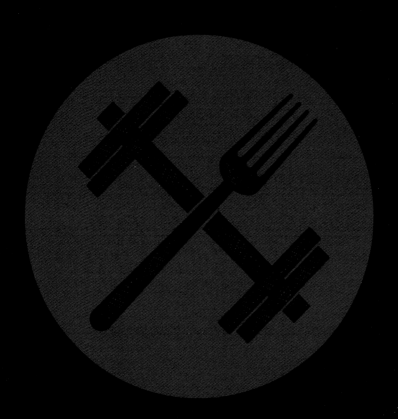

CLEAN SIMPLE EATS

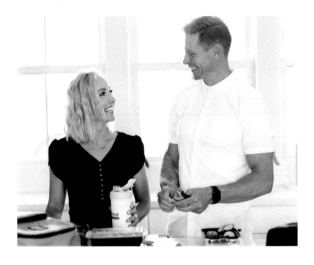

We have been creating and testing these Clean Simple Treats in our own kitchen for years and we are so excited to share the love with you! We have put a healthier spin on all of our favorite dessert recipes without sacrificing any of the flavor! You can now have your cake and eat it too! We hope these recipes become staples in your home like they have in ours.

Enjoy! XO Erika & JJ

STAY CONNECTED

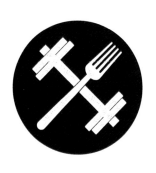

 @cleansimpleeats

 facebook.com/groups/cleansimpleeats

 hello@cleansimpleeats.com

 www.cleansimpleeats.com

For a list of cookie scoops we use, pans we love, and where to purchase some of the harder to find ingredients found in this book, visit our website: cleansimpleeats.com/products-we-love.

RECIPE INDEX

BREADS & ROLLS

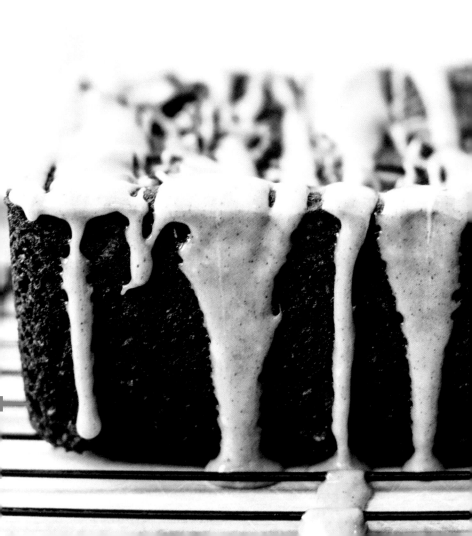

GOOD THINGS COME TO THOSE WHO BAKE

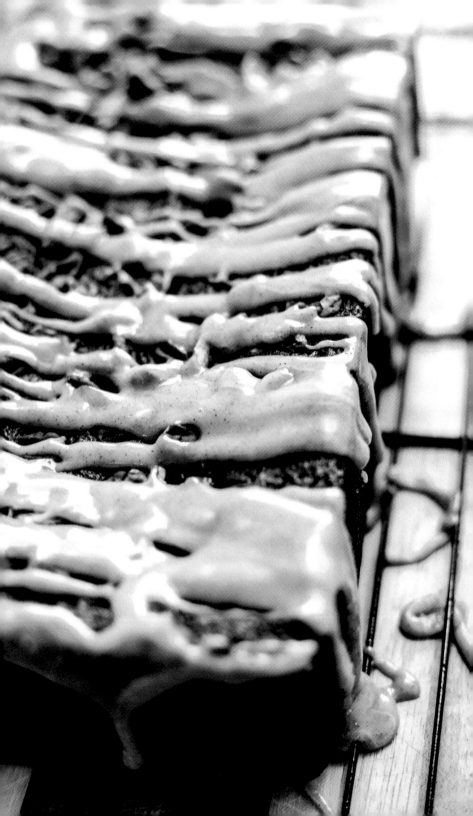

CARAMEL-GLAZED PUMPKIN PECAN BREAD

Makes 2 loaves / 10 slices per loaf
285 calories / 11F / 40C / 7P / per slice

---

1 cup raw honey
1 cup coconut sugar
½ cup melted coconut oil
1 cup canned pumpkin
½ cup unsweetened applesauce
4 large eggs
⅔ cup water
3 ½ cups Kodiak Cakes Buttermilk Mix
2 tsp. baking soda
1 tsp. ground cinnamon
1 tsp. ground nutmeg
½ tsp. sea salt
½ cup chopped pecans
Caramel Sauce:
¼ cup OffBeat Salted Caramel Butter, Pumpkin Spice Butter,
    Butter Pecan Pie Butter, or natural almond butter
¼ cup raw honey
½ tsp. vanilla extract
Dash of sea salt

1. Preheat oven to 350 degrees.

2. Beat the honey, coconut sugar and coconut oil together in a bowl. Beat in the pumpkin, applesauce, eggs and water; set aside.

3. In a separate bowl, mix together Kodiak Cakes, baking soda, cinnamon, nutmeg and sea salt. Add wet ingredients to the dry ingredients and mix until just combined.

4. Pour the batter evenly into two greased, 9x5 inch, glass loaf pans and then sprinkle ¼ cup of the chopped pecans over the top of each loaf. Bake for 45 minutes or until golden on top and fully cooked through. Let cool for 20 minutes, then transfer to a plate or cooling rack.

5. Make the caramel sauce by adding all the caramel ingredients to a small saucepan over low heat. Stir constantly until completely melted and pourable. Drizzle the caramel sauce evenly over the two loaves and then let cool. Slice and enjoy!

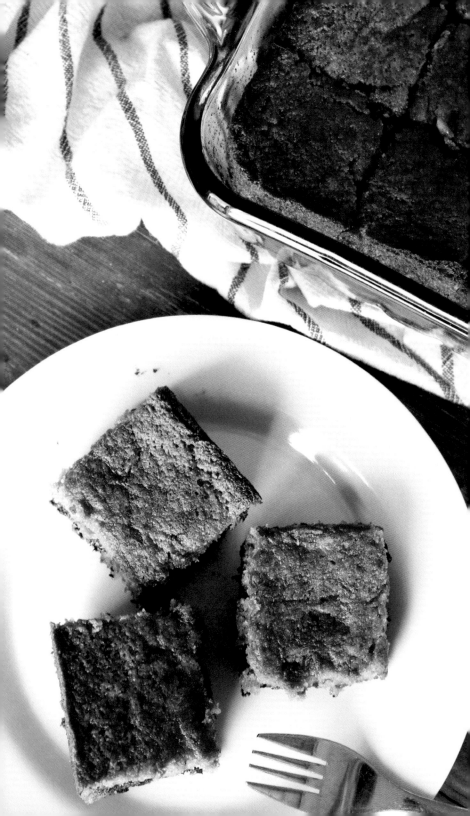

CHOCOLATE CHIP BANANA BREAD SQUARES

Makes 16 servings
145 calories / 5F / 22C / 3.5P / per square

---

2 ripe bananas
½ cup unsweetened applesauce
3 Tbs. melted coconut oil
½ cup raw honey
1 large egg
1 tsp. vanilla extract
1 ½ cups Kodiak Cakes Buttermilk Mix
1 tsp. baking soda
½ tsp. ground cinnamon
¼ tsp. sea salt
½ cup dark chocolate chips

1. Preheat oven to 350 degrees.

2. Mash the bananas in a large bowl. Beat in the applesauce, coconut oil and honey. Add the egg and vanilla; mix well.

3. In a separate bowl, combine the Kodiak Cakes Mix, baking soda, cinnamon and sea salt. Add the dry ingredients to the wet ingredients and mix until just combined.

4. Pour the mixture into a greased, 8x8 baking pan. Sprinkle the chocolate chips on top. Bake for 40 minutes, then let cool. Cut into 16 squares. Enjoy!

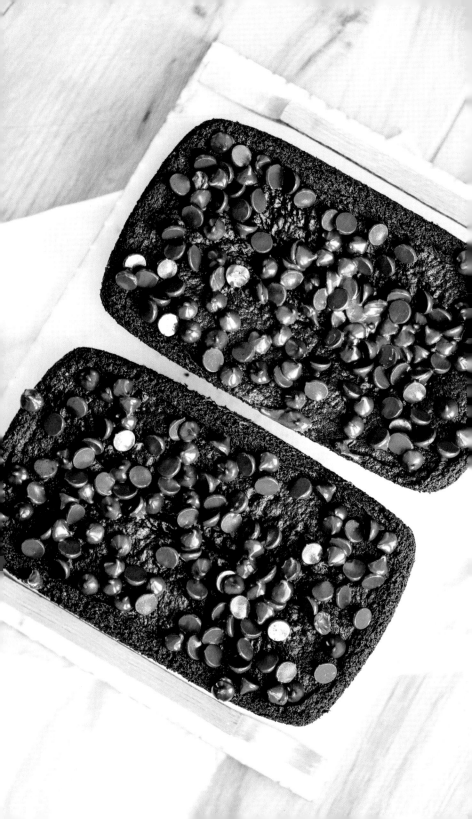

DOUBLE CHOCOLATE BANANA BREAD

Makes 1 loaf / 10 slices
265 calories / 10.5F / 36C / 6.5P / per slice

---

3 ripe bananas
½ cup unsweetened applesauce
½ cup raw honey
¼ cup melted coconut oil
1 large egg
1 tsp. vanilla extract
1 cup Kodiak Cakes Buttermilk Mix
1 serving CSE Brownie Batter Protein Powder
⅓ cup cocoa powder
1 tsp. baking soda
½ tsp. sea salt
½ cup dark chocolate chips

1. Preheat oven to 350 degrees.

2. Mash the bananas in a large bowl. Beat in the applesauce, honey and melted coconut oil. Add the egg and vanilla; mix well.

3. In a separate bowl combine the Kodiak Cakes, protein powder, cocoa powder, baking soda and sea salt. Add the dry ingredients to the wet ingredients. Mix until just combined.

4. Pour into a greased, 9x5 inch, glass loaf pan and sprinkle with the chocolate chips. Bake for 50-55 minutes, then let cool. Remove from the pan and drizzle with extra melted chocolate, if desired. Enjoy!!

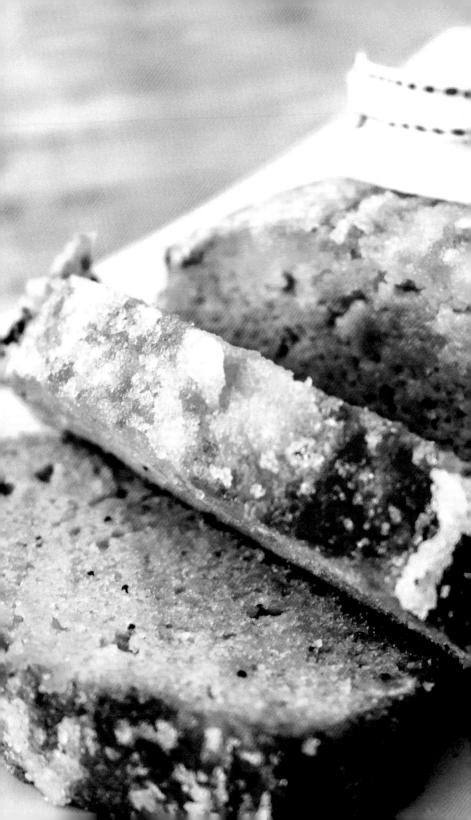

ORANGE-GLAZED CHIA SEED BREAD

Makes 1 loaf / 10 slices
230 calories / 4F / 44C / 5P / per slice

1 cup white whole wheat flour
1 serving CSE Simply Vanilla Protein Powder
1 Tbs. chia seeds
½ tsp. sea salt
½ tsp. baking powder
1 large egg
¾ cup raw honey
½ cup unsweetened almond milk
¼ cup unsweetened applesauce
2 Tbs. melted coconut oil
1 tsp. melted grass-fed butter
½ tsp. vanilla extract
½ tsp. almond extract
Glaze:
1 cup powdered sugar
2 Tbs. pasteurized egg whites
1 Tbs. fresh squeezed orange juice
1 tsp. orange zest

1. Preheat oven to 350 degrees.

2. Mix the the flour, protein powder, chia seeds, sea salt and baking powder in a bowl; set aside.

3. In a separate bowl beat the egg, honey, almond milk, applesauce, coconut oil, butter, vanilla extract and almond extract. Add the dry ingredients to the wet ingredients and mix on low until just combined.

4. Pour into a greased, 9x5 inch, glass loaf pan. Bake for 40-45 minutes or until golden on the top and cooked through. Let cool.

5. Beat together all the glaze ingredients until smooth. Once the bread is cooled, drizzle the glaze over the top of the bread and store in the fridge. Slice and enjoy!

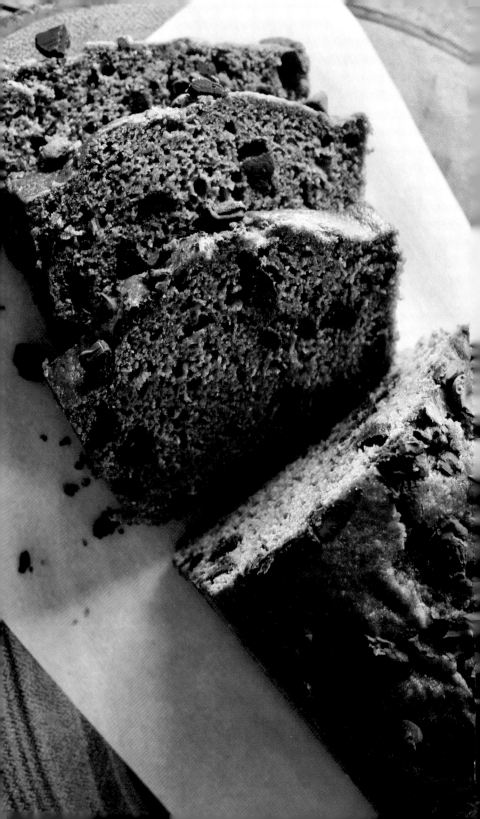

PUMPKIN CHOCOLATE CHIP BREAD

Makes 2 loaves / 10 slices per loaf
210 calories / 4.5F / 37C / 5P / per slice

---

15 oz. canned pumpkin
3 large eggs
¾ cup raw honey
¾ cup coconut sugar
½ cup unsweetened applesauce
½ cup nonfat, plain Greek yogurt
2 Tbs. fresh squeezed orange juice
½ Tbs. molasses
1 tsp. vanilla extract
3 cups white whole wheat flour
2 tsp. ground cinnamon
½ tsp. ground nutmeg
½ tsp. ground cloves
1 tsp. baking powder
1 tsp. baking soda
½ tsp. sea salt
1 cup dark chocolate chips

1. Preheat oven to 350 degrees.

2. Beat the pumpkin, eggs, honey, coconut sugar, applesauce, Greek yogurt, orange juice, molasses and vanilla together in a large bowl. Mix until well combined; set aside.

3. In a separate bowl, stir the flour, cinnamon, nutmeg, cloves, baking powder, baking soda and sea salt together. Add the wet ingredients to the dry ingredients and stir until just combined. Stir in ⅔ cup of the chocolate chips.

4. Grease two, 9x5 inch, glass loaf pans. Pour the batter evenly into the two pans then sprinkle the remaining ⅓ cup chocolate chips over the top.

5. Bake for 40 minutes. Remove from the oven and cover loosely with foil. Bake an additional 10 minutes and let cool. Enjoy!

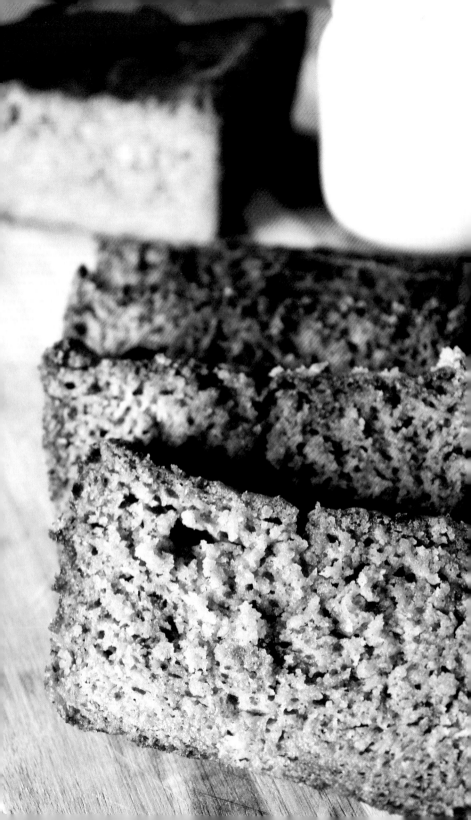

SIMPLE BANANA BREAD

Makes 2 loaves / 10 slices per loaf
180 calories / 5F / 28C / 5.5P / per slice

---

4 ripe bananas
6 Tbs. softened butter or coconut oil
1 cup unsweetened applesauce
½ cup raw honey
½ cup coconut sugar
2 large eggs
2 tsp. vanilla extract
3 cups Kodiak Cakes Buttermilk Mix
1 tsp. baking soda
1 tsp. ground cinnamon
½ tsp. sea salt

1. Preheat oven to 350 degrees.

2. Mash the bananas in a bowl. Beat in the butter/coconut oil, applesauce, honey and coconut sugar. Add eggs and vanilla. Beat on high until well combined.

3. In a separate bowl, combine the Kodiak Cakes Mix, baking soda, cinnamon and sea salt. Add the dry mixture to the wet mixture. Stir slowly until just combined.

4. Grease two, 9x5 inch loaf pans. Pour mixture evenly into both pans and bake for 50 minutes. Check the bread at 30 minutes. If the bread is getting too dark on the top, lightly place a sheet of foil over the top for the remaining time. Let cool. Enjoy!

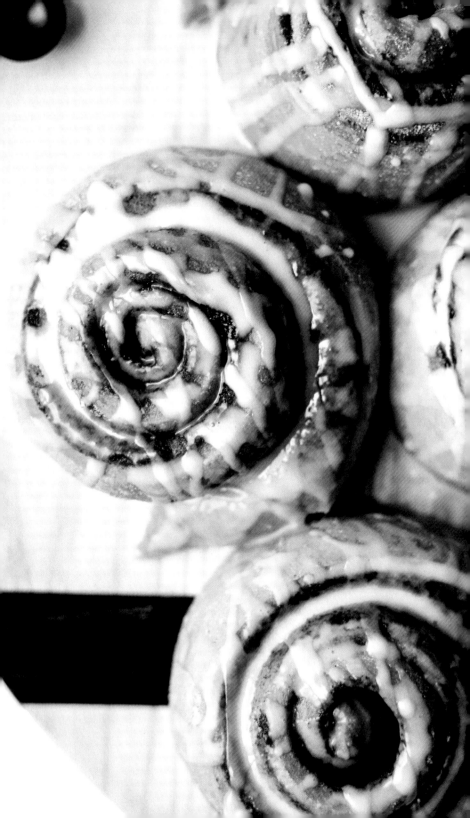

SWEET HONEY CINNAMON ROLLS

Makes 24 rolls
185 calories / 6F / 29C / 4P / per roll with icing

2 large eggs
2 ½ tsp. instant yeast
½ cup warm water (100-115 degrees)
1 cup cooked, peeled & mashed sweet potatoes
1 cup unsweetened almond milk
½ cup cold grass-fed butter
½ cup raw honey
1 tsp. sea salt
5 cups white whole wheat flour
Filling:
2 Tbs. melted grass-fed butter
2 Tbs. coconut sugar
1 Tbs. ground cinnamon
Icing:
1 cup powdered sugar
2 Tbs. pasteurized egg whites
¼ tsp. butter extract

1. Beat eggs in a small bowl; set aside. In a separate bowl, dissolve yeast into warm water. Once dissolved, pour eggs into water with yeast; set aside. Remove the skins from the cooked sweet potatoes and beat with hand mixers until smooth; set aside.

2. Heat almond milk in a pot over high heat until small bubbles form around the edges. Remove from heat. Add the cold butter, honey, salt and sweet potatoes. Stir until all the butter is melted and the mixture is smooth.

3. Place in a bread or Kitchen Aid mixer. Add the egg mixture and the flour. Knead for 10 minutes. Cover and let rise in the fridge for 2 hours.

4. Split the dough in half. Place the dough on a floured surface and roll both pieces into large, thin rectangles. Mix the filling ingredients together and then spread evenly all over dough. Slice each rectangle into 12 strips and roll up. Place on a greased baking sheet; 12 rolls per sheet. Cover with a dish towel and let rise for 5+ hours or overnight.

5. Bake at 375 degrees for 12 minutes or until lightly browned. Beat icing ingredients together and drizzle over the top. Enjoy!

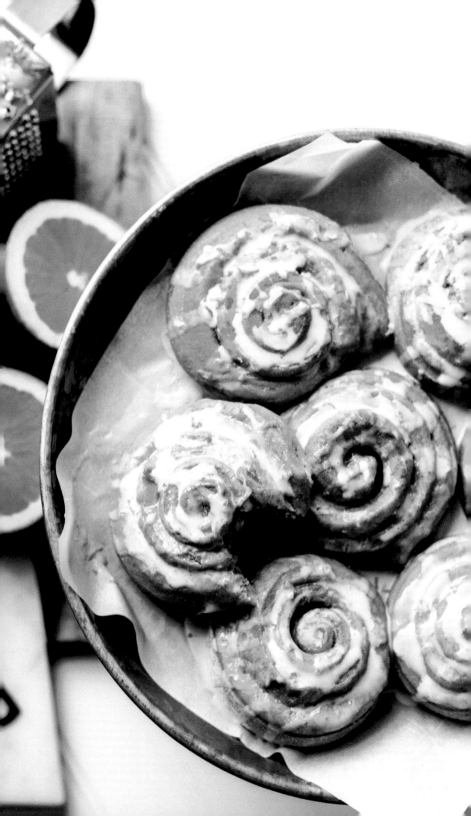

ZESTY ORANGE SWEET ROLLS

Makes 24 rolls
185 calories / 6F / 29C / 4P / per roll with glaze

2 large eggs
2 ½ tsp. instant yeast
½ cup warm water (100-115 degrees)
1 cup cooked, peeled & mashed sweet potatoes
1 cup unsweetened almond milk
½ cup cold grass-fed butter
½ cup raw honey
1 tsp. sea salt
5 cups white whole wheat flour

Filling:
2 Tbs. melted grass-fed butter
2 Tbs. raw honey
1 tsp. orange zest

Glaze:
1 cup powdered sugar
2 Tbs. pasteurized egg whites
1 Tbs. fresh squeezed orange juice
1 tsp. orange zest

1. Beat eggs in a small bowl; set aside. In a separate bowl, dissolve yeast into warm water. Once dissolved, pour eggs into water with yeast; set aside. Remove the skins from the sweet potatoes and beat with hand mixers until smooth; set aside.

2. Heat almond milk in a pot over high heat until small bubbles form around the edges. Remove from heat. Add the cold butter, honey, salt and sweet potatoes. Stir until all the butter is melted and the mixture is smooth.

3. Place in a bread or Kitchen Aid mixer. Add the egg mixture and the flour. Knead for 10 minutes. Cover and let rise in the fridge for 2 hours.

4. Split the dough in half. Place the dough on a floured surface and roll both pieces into large, thin rectangles. Mix the filling ingredients together and then spread evenly all over dough. Slice each rectangle into 12 strips and roll up. Place on a greased baking sheet; 12 rolls per sheet. Cover with a dish towel and let rise for 5+ hours or overnight.

5. Bake at 375 degrees for 12 minutes or until lightly browned. Beat glaze ingredients together and drizzle over the top. Enjoy!

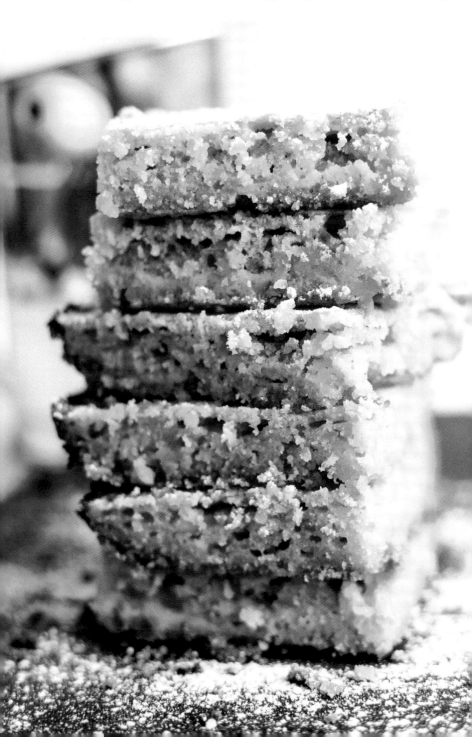

BROWNIES & BARS

DESSERT IS LIKE A FEEL GOOD SONG AND THE BEST ONES MAKE YOU DANCE

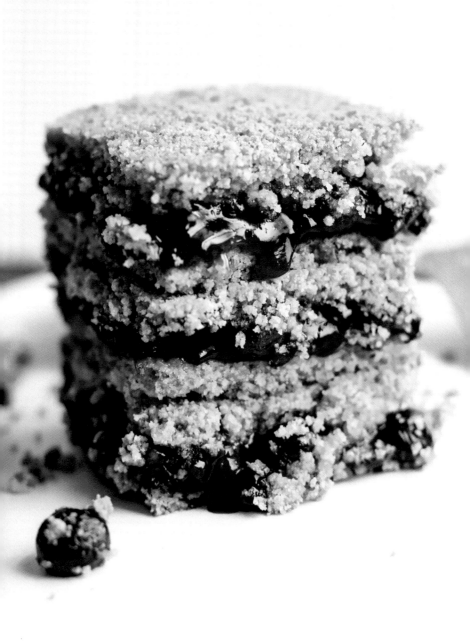

BLUEBERRY CRUMBLE BARS

Makes 18 bars
215 calories / 9F / 29C / 5P / per bar

Crust/Topping:
¾ cup xylitol sweetener
¼ cup coconut sugar
3 cups Kodiak Cakes Buttermilk Mix
¼ tsp. sea salt
1 lemon, zest of
¾ cup grass-fed butter
¼ cup flaxseed meal
1 large egg
Filling:
1 Tbs. cornstarch or arrowroot powder
2 Tbs. water
¼ cup xylitol sweetener
¼ cup raw honey
4 cups fresh blueberries

1. Preheat oven to 375 degrees.

2. Stir together the xylitol, coconut sugar, Kodiak Cakes Mix, sea salt and lemon zest in a bowl. Add the butter, flaxseed meal and egg. Stir together until the mixture begins to ball. Split the mixture in half and press one half of it into the bottom of a greased 9x13 baking pan.

3. Make the filling: In a small bowl, dissolve the cornstarch or arrow-root powder into the water. Add that mixture to a sauce pan over low heat with the xylitol and honey; whisk until smooth. Add the blueber-ries to the pan. Turn the heat up to high and bring to a boil, stirring constantly with a rubber spatula. Remove from heat and continue to stir as the sauce thickens. Pour the blueberry mixture evenly over the top of the crust and then sprinkle the remaining crumble mixture over the top and press down to cover the blueberry filling.

4. Bake for 20-25 minutes or until the top is golden brown. Let cool completely and then cut into bars. Enjoy as is or topped with spray whipped cream or ice cream. Enjoy!

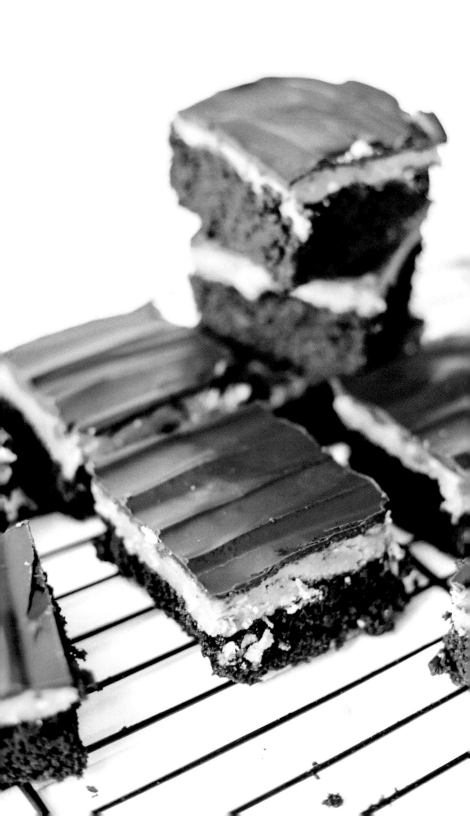

BUCKEYE BROWNIES

Makes 20 servings
390 calories / 18F / 51C / 6P / per brownie

1 ⅓ cups raw honey
1 cup unsweetened applesauce
¼ cup light-tasting olive oil
6 Tbs. liquid egg whites
2 tsp. vanilla extract
⅔ cup cocoa powder
1 cup white whole wheat flour
½ tsp. sea salt
½ tsp. baking soda
½ tsp. baking powder

Peanut Butter Cream:
½ cup coconut oil or grass-fed butter
1 cup OffBeat Sweet Classic Peanut Butter, Buckeye Brownie Peanut Butter,
    or creamy natural peanut butter
2 cups Swerve Confectioners Sweetener
1 tsp. vanilla extract
2 Tbs. full-fat coconut milk
Dash of sea salt

Chocolate Topping:
1 cup dark chocolate chips, melted

1. Preheat oven to 350 degrees.

2. Beat the honey, applesauce, olive oil, egg whites and vanilla together in a bowl; set aside.

3. In a separate bowl, combine the cocoa powder, flour, sea salt, baking soda and baking powder together. Add the dry ingredients to the wet ingredients and mix until just combined. Pour the batter into a greased 9x13 baking dish and bake for 25 minutes. Place in the fridge on a heating pad to cool.

4. Make the peanut butter cream: Beat the butter or coconut oil together with the peanut butter. Slowly beat in the Swerve sweetener until well combined. Mix in the vanilla, coconut milk and sea salt. Spread over the cooled brownies and place in the fridge for 30 minutes before adding the chocolate topping.

5. Place the chocolate chips in a bowl and melt in the microwave. Heat 30 seconds at a time until melted and smooth, stirring in between. Drizzle the melted chocolate over the top of the brownies and spread evenly.

6. Let sit in the fridge for one hour before serving. Cut into 20 brownies. Enjoy!

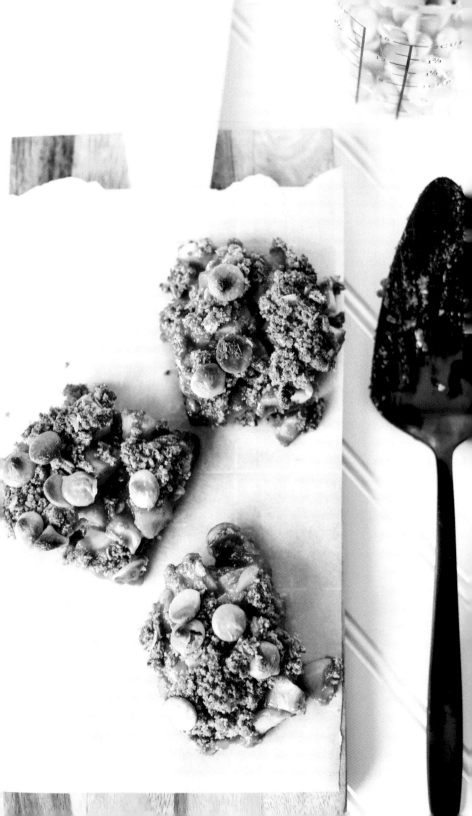

CARAMEL APPLE BARS
Makes 18 bars
305 calories / 14F / 36C / 9P / per bar

½ cup + 2 Tbs. grass-fed butter
2 Tbs. flaxseed meal
¾ cup coconut sugar
1 large egg
1 tsp. vanilla extract
1 ¾ cup Kodiak Cakes Cinnamon Oat Mix
1 cup old-fashioned rolled oats
½ tsp. sea salt
½ tsp. baking soda
Filling:
2 Tbs. grass-fed butter
4 cups chopped apples
½ cup OffBeat Salted Caramel Butter, Cinnamon Bun Butter,
    or natural almond butter
½ cup raw honey
½ cup caramel flavored chips

1. Preheat oven to 400 degrees.

2. Beat the butter, flaxseed meal, coconut sugar, egg and vanilla together in a large bowl. Add the Kodiak Cakes Mix, rolled oats, sea salt and baking soda; mix well. Split the crumble mixture in half.

3. Press one half of the crumble into the bottom of a greased 9x13 baking pan; set aside.

4. Make the filling: In a sauce pan, melt the butter over low heat. Stir the chopped apples into the melted butter and sauté for 1-2 minutes. Add in the nut butter and honey. Mix until completely melted and apples are well coated. Pour the apple mixture evenly over the crust. Sprinkle the caramel chips over the apples and then top with the remaining crumble mixture.

5. Bake for 15-20 minutes or until the top is lightly browned. Let cool, then cut into bars. Enjoy as is or top with spray whipped cream or ice cream.

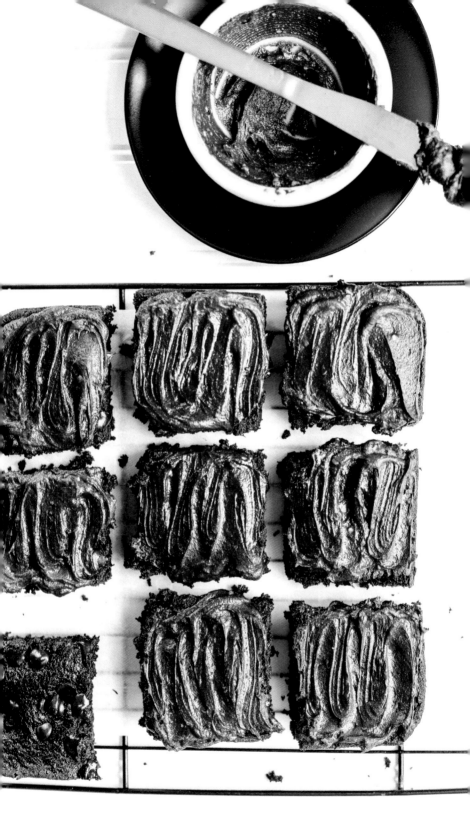

CHOVOCADO BROWNIES

Makes 12 brownies
180 calories / 6.5F / 27C / 4P / per brownie

⅔ cup raw honey
⅓ cup cocoa powder
½ cup unsweetened applesauce
1 tsp. vanilla extract
2 Tbs. light-tasting olive oil
1 large egg
½ cup white whole wheat flour
1 Tbs. flaxseed meal
¼ tsp. baking soda
¼ tsp. baking powder
¼ tsp. sea salt
¼ cup dark chocolate chips

Chovocado Frosting:
¼ (25g) of a ripe avocado
2 Tbs. OffBeat Sweet Classic Peanut Butter, Midnight Almond
    Coconut Butter, Buckeye Brownie Peanut Butter,
    or natural almond butter
2 Tbs. cocoa powder
1 serving CSE Brownie Batter Protein Powder
¼ cup unsweetened almond milk
1 Tbs. raw honey

1. Preheat oven to 350 degrees.

2. Heat the honey in the microwave for 45 seconds. Stir the cocoa powder into the honey until completely dissolved; set aside.

3. In a separate bowl, beat the applesauce, vanilla, olive oil and egg together. Add the chocolate/honey mixture to the bowl; mix well. Add the flour, flaxseed meal, baking soda, baking powder and sea salt to the bowl and mix until just combined.

4. Pour the batter into a greased 8x8 baking dish. Sprinkle the chocolate chips over the top. Bake for 25 minutes, then let cool.

5. Beat all of the frosting ingredients together in a bowl. Once the brownies are cooled off, spread the frosting over the top and slice into 12 servings. Enjoy!

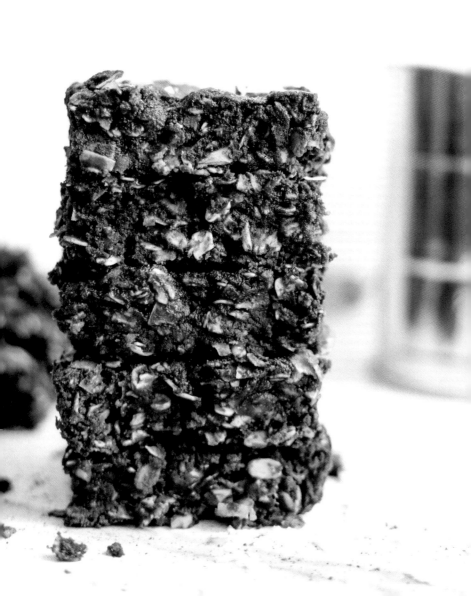

COCOA PEANUT BUTTER BARS

Makes 18 Bars
240 calories / 11F / 28C / 7P / per bar

1 cup OffBeat Sweet Classic Peanut Butter,
    Buckeye Brownie Peanut Butter, or natural peanut butter
1 cup raw honey
2 large eggs
1 ⅓ cups unsweetened applesauce
2 cups old-fashioned rolled oats
1 serving CSE Brownie Batter Protein Powder
½ cup cocoa powder
½ cup almond flour
½ cup unsweetened coconut flakes

1. Preheat oven to 375 degrees.

2. Beat the peanut butter, honey, eggs and applesauce together in a bowl; set aside.

3. Add the remaining dry ingredients to a separate bowl. Stir until well combined. Add the wet ingredients to the dry ingredients. Mix until just combined.

4. Pour the batter into a greased 9x13 pan. Bake for 15-20 minutes. Let cool and then cut into 18 squares. Enjoy!

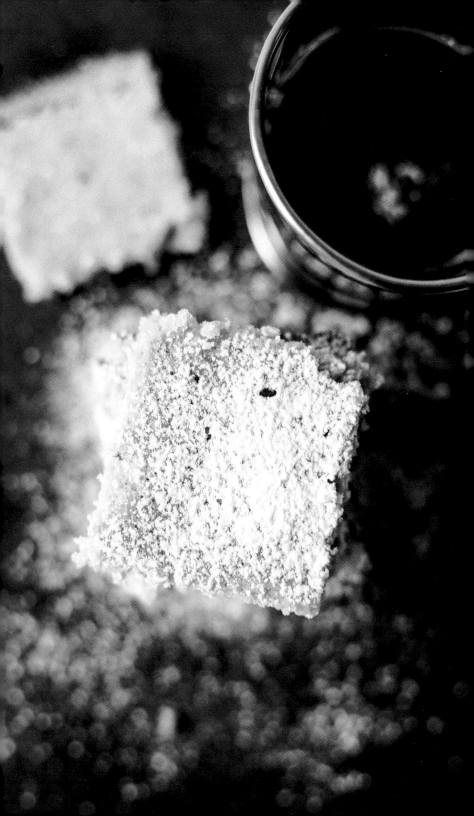

LEMON MACADAMIA BARS
Makes 18 bars
165 calories / 7F / 21C / 5P / per bar

Crust:
½ cup Kodiak Cakes Buttermilk Mix
½ cup macadamia nuts, finely chopped
¼ cup CSE Simply Vanilla or Coconut Cream Protein Powder
½ cup softened OffBeat Lemon Coconut Bliss Butter,
    coconut butter, or coconut manna

Filling:
2 large eggs
4 egg whites
¼ cup Kodiak Cakes Buttermilk Mix
½ tsp. baking powder
1 cup raw honey
2 lemons, juice of
1 lemon, zest of

Topping:
¼ cup powdered sugar (optional garnish)

1. Preheat oven to 350 degrees.

2. Combine all the crust ingredients together and press into the bottom of a greased 9x13 baking pan. Bake for 15 minutes. Remove from the oven and let cool.

3. In a large bowl, beat the eggs and eggs whites together. Add the Kodiak Cakes Mix, baking powder, honey, lemon juice and lemon zest. Pour over the top of the crust. Bake for 20-25 minutes or until the edges are golden brown and the mixture is set.

4. Let the bars cool, then cut into squares. Sprinkle powdered sugar over the top and serve. Enjoy!

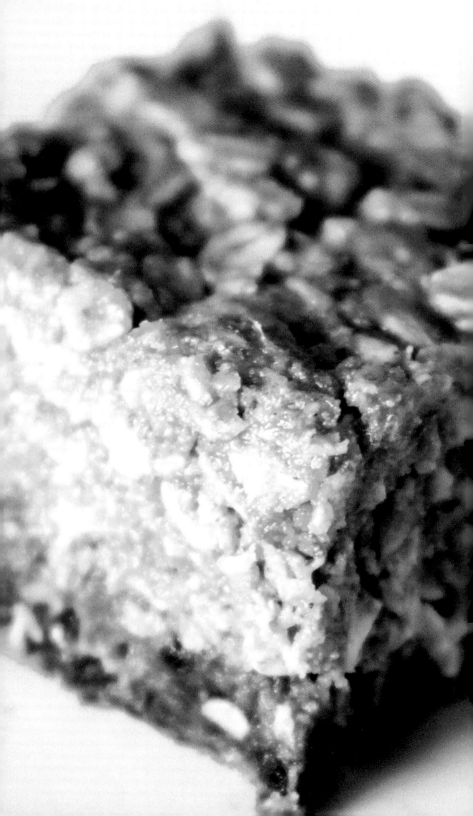

PUMPKIN PIE NO-BAKE BARS

Makes 18 servings
325 calories / 12F / 48C / 6P / per bar

Crust:
1 cup raw almonds
½ tsp. sea salt
40 dates, pitted
¼ cup unsweetened almond milk
Bar:
1 cup raw honey
½ cup coconut sugar
½ cup melted coconut oil
¾ cup canned pumpkin
1 tsp. vanilla extract
1 tsp. pumpkin pie spice
3 ½ cups old-fashioned rolled oats
¼ cup flaxseed meal
1 serving CSE Simply Vanilla
    or Pumpkin Pie Protein Powder

1. Pulse the almonds and salt in a high-powered blender until finely chopped. Pour into a bowl and set aside. Add the dates and almond milk to the blender. Pulse until it turns into a paste. Pour into the bowl with the almonds and mix well.

2. Press the mixture into a greased 9x13 pan and place in the freezer. Let harden until finished with the next step.

3. Beat the honey, coconut sugar and melted coconut oil together in a bowl. Add the pumpkin, vanilla extract, pumpkin pie spice, rolled oats, flaxseed meal and protein powder. Mix until well combined.

4. Pour the pumpkin mixture into the 9x13 pan over the crust. Freeze 4+ hours. Cut into 18 bars and serve cold. Enjoy!

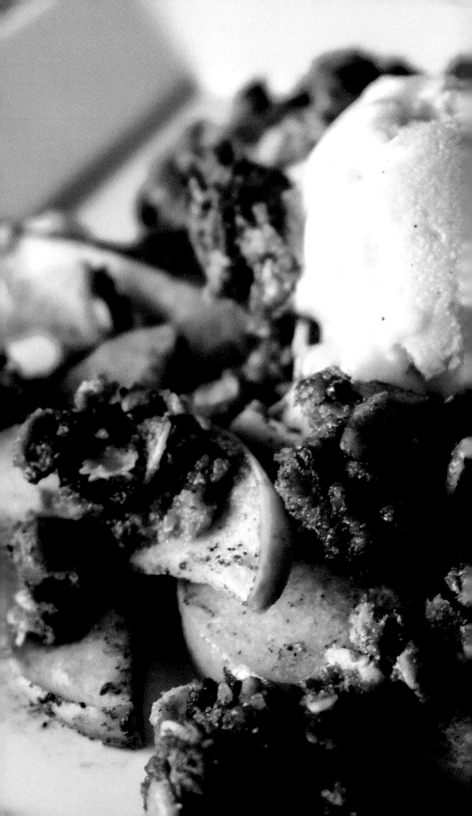

PUMPKIN-SPICED APPLE CRISP

Makes 12 servings
250 calories / 9.5F / 35C / 6.5P / per serving w/o topping

1 cup old-fashioned rolled oats
1 cup Kodiak Cakes Cinnamon Oat Mix
1 cup coconut sugar
¼ cup chopped pecans
1 tsp. pumpkin pie spice
Pinch of sea salt
7 Tbs. softened grass-fed butter
3 Tbs. canned pumpkin
4 medium-sized apples
½ tsp. ground cinnamon
Optional toppings:
Protein-packed ice cream
Spray whipped cream

1. Preheat oven to 325 degrees.

2. In a large bowl stir together the rolled oats, Kodiak Cakes Mix, coconut sugar, chopped pecans, pumpkin pie spice and sea salt; set aside.

3. Beat six tablespoons of the butter and the canned pumpkin together. Stir into the dry mix until it becomes crumbly; set aside.

4. Peel and thinly slice the apples. Add the remaining tablespoon of butter to a large saute pan and melt over low/medium heat. Once melted, add the apples and cinnamon. Stir together and cook for three minutes. Pour into a greased 9x13 baking dish, then sprinkle the crumble mixture over the top.

5. Bake for 40-45 minutes, then let cool. Enjoy warm topped with ice cream or spray whipped cream.

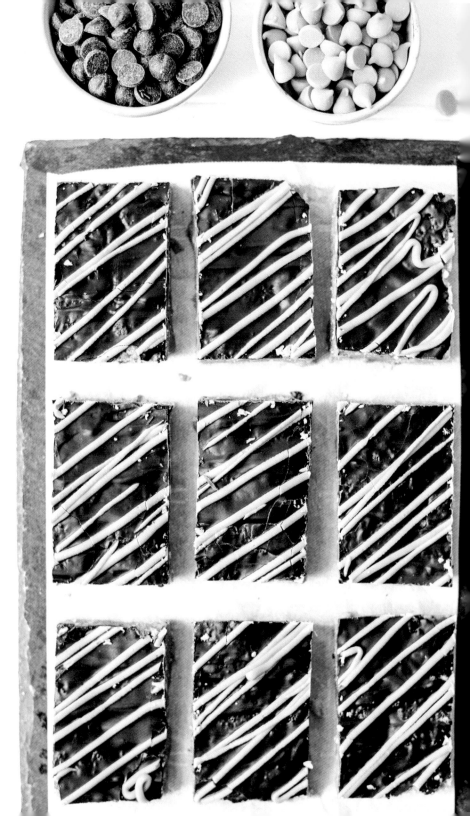

SCOTCHAROO BARS

Makes 18 bars
255 calories / 12.5F / 28.5C / 7.5P / per bar

1 cup OffBeat Sweet Classic Peanut Butter,
   Candy Bar Butter, or natural peanut butter
1 cup powdered peanut butter
¾ cup raw honey
¼ cup flaxseed meal
2 Tbs. unsweetened almond milk
1 tsp. vanilla extract
¼ tsp. sea salt
1 serving CSE Simply Vanilla Protein Powder
¼ cup butterscotch chips
2 cups Rice Krispies cereal

Toppings:
¼ cup butterscotch chips
½ cup dark chocolate chips

1. Mix the peanut butter, powdered peanut butter, honey, flaxseed meal, almond milk, vanilla extract, sea salt and protein powder together in a bowl. Melt ¼ cup of the butterscotch chips and mix in. Add the Rice Krispies cereal last and gently mix until well combined. Press into a 9x13 pan; set aside.

2. Place the chocolate chips in a bowl and microwave 30 seconds at a time until completely melted and smooth, stirring in between. Drizzle over the top of the bars and spread out smooth. Melt the remaining ¼ cup of butterscotch chips and drizzle over the top of the chocolate.

3. Store in the fridge for 1 hour to allow the chocolate to harden. Cut into 18 bars. Enjoy!

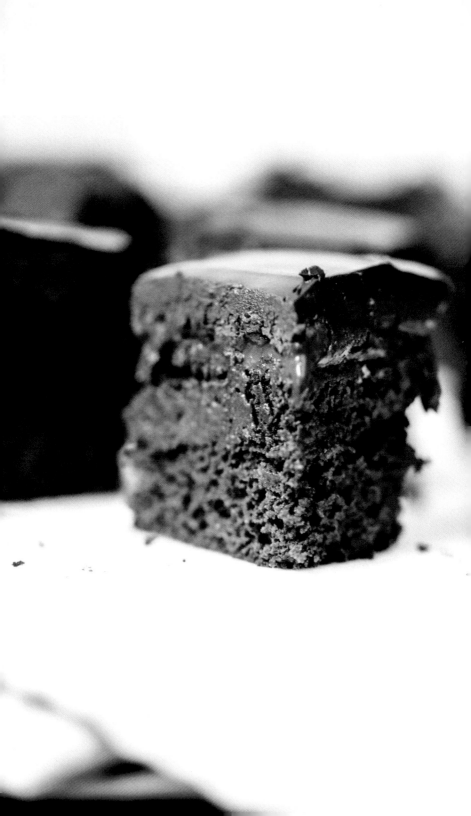

THIN MINT CHOCOLATE BROWNIES

Makes 36 brownies
100 calories / 4.5F / 12C / 2.5P / per brownie

¾ cup oat flour
½ cup cocoa powder
1 serving CSE Brownie Batter
    or Mint Chocolate Cookie Protein Powder
½ tsp. baking powder
⅛ tsp. sea salt
2 Tbs. grass-fed butter
½ cup raw honey
1 large egg
2 egg whites
½ cup unsweetened applesauce
1 Tbs. vanilla extract

Toppings:
1 cup OffBeat Mint Chocolate Chip Cookie Butter
2 Tbs. grass-fed butter
½ cup dark chocolate chips

1. Preheat oven to 350 degrees.

2. Stir the dry ingredients together in a small bowl; set aside.

3. In a separate bowl, beat the butter and honey together. Add the eggs, egg whites, applesauce and vanilla; mix well. Add the wet ingredients to the dry ingredients and mix until just combined.

4. Pour into a greased 8x8 glass baking dish. Bake for 20-25 minutes, then let cool.

5. Once the brownies are cool, pour softened OffBeat Butter over the top and spread out evenly. Place in the freezer until the chocolate has set.

6. Place the butter and chocolate chips in a bowl. Microwave 30 seconds at a time until melted and smooth, stirring in between. Pour over the brownies and spread out smooth. Return to the fridge or freezer for about 1 hour or until the chocolate has set. Allow brownies to sit out at room temperature for about 5-10 minutes before slicing. Slice into 36 brownie bites and enjoy!

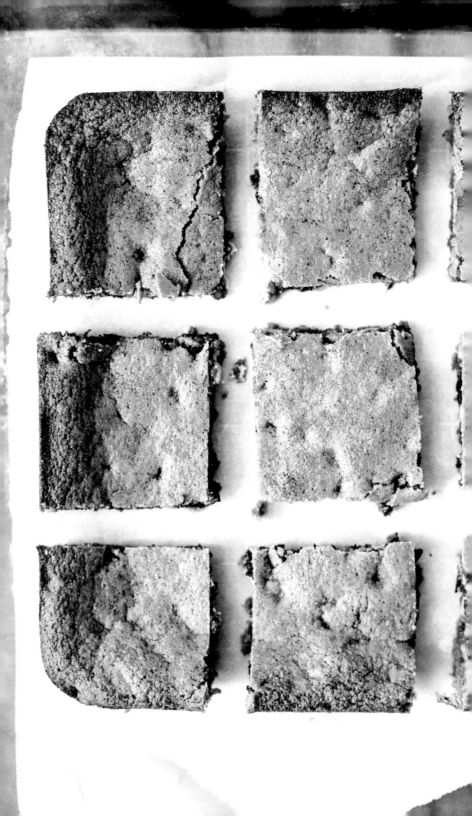

TRIPLE CHIP BLONDIES

Makes 18 bars
270 calories / 12F / 36C / 4P / per bar

½ cup grass-fed butter
1 cup xylitol sweetener
1 cup coconut sugar
2 large eggs
1 Tbs. vanilla extract
2 cups Kodiak Cakes Buttermilk Mix
Pinch of sea salt
1 tsp. baking powder
½ cup butterscotch chips
¼ cup white or vanilla chocolate chips
¼ cup dark chocolate chips

1. Preheat oven to 350 degrees.

2. Beat the butter, xylitol and coconut sugar together in a bowl. Add the eggs and vanilla and beat until well combined; set aside.

3. In a separate bowl, stir together the Kodiak Cakes Mix, sea salt and baking powder. Add the wet ingredients to the dry ingredients and mix until just combined. Fold in all the chips.

4. Press the dough into a greased 9x13 baking pan and bake for 20-25 minutes or until golden brown. Let cool, then slice into 18 bars. Enjoy!

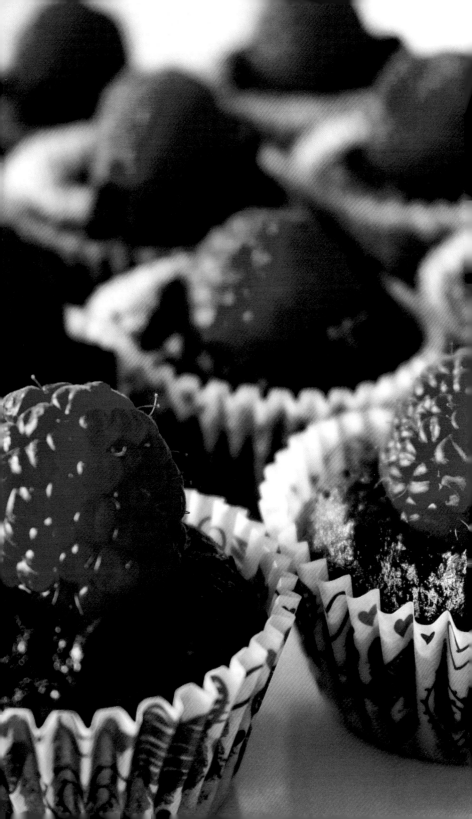

TWO-BITE BROWNIES

Makes 12 brownies
130 calories / 5F / 18C / 3P / per brownie

1 large egg
½ cup raw honey
¼ cup OffBeat Midnight Almond Coconut Butter,
    Buckeye Brownie Peanut Butter, or natural almond butter
2 Tbs. unsweetened almond milk
⅓ cup cocoa powder
½ serving CSE Brownie Batter Protein Powder
½ tsp. sea salt
¼ cup mini chocolate chips
12 raspberries

1. Preheat oven to 350 degrees.

2. Beat the egg, honey, nut butter and almond milk together in a bowl. Add the cocoa powder, protein powder, sea salt and mini chocolate chips; mix well.

3. Place mini muffin liners in a mini muffin pan. Spray liners with cooking spray and add brownie batter to the muffin liners. Fill each liner ¾ full with batter.

4. Bake for 8-10 minutes; they should still be gooey in the middle. Press one raspberry on the top of each brownie bite. Store in the fridge or freezer. Enjoy hot or cold!

CAKES

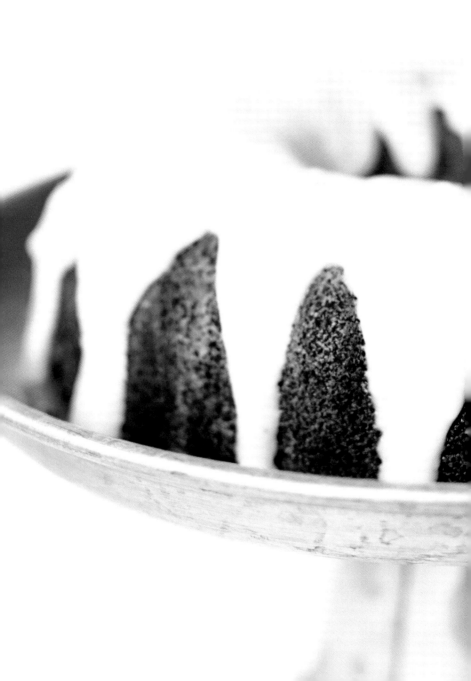

A PARTY WITHOUT CAKE IS JUST A MEETING

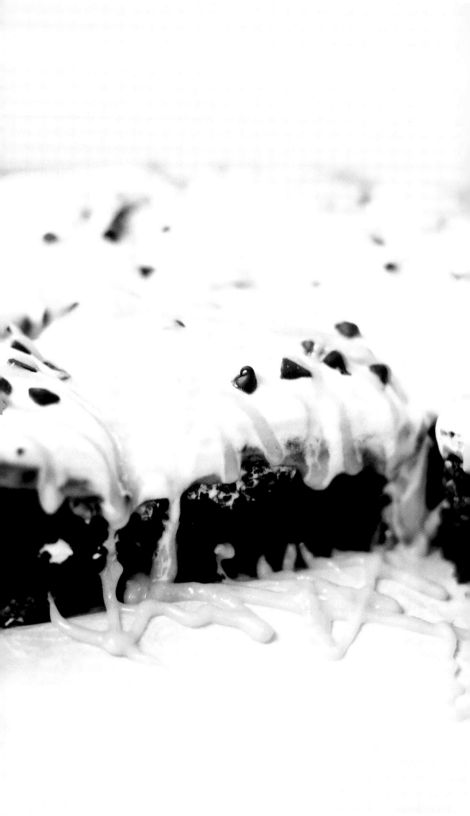

BETTER THAN JUNK FOOD CAKE

Makes 18 servings
325 calories / 16F / 39C / 6.5P / per serving

CSE Devil's Food Cake Recipe (page 55)
Caramel Sauce Filling:
½ cup Cashew Coconut Caramel Sauce (recipe below)
¼ cup caramel flavored chips
Coconut Cream:
2 cups coconut milk, full-fat
⅓ cup Swerve Confectioners Sweetener
1 tsp. vanilla extract
Topping:
½ cup mini chocolate chips
Caramel Sauce Topping:
¼ cup Cashew Coconut Caramel Sauce
¼ cup caramel flavored chips

1. Place your coconut milk in the fridge (do not shake) to firm up for 1+ hours.

2. Make the CSE Devil's Food Cake recipe. Poke holes all over, halfway down into the cake. Let cool slightly while making the caramel sauce filling.

3. Make the caramel sauce filling by placing ½ cup of the Cashew Coconut Caramel Sauce and ¼ cup caramel chips in a saucepan over low heat. Stir continuously until well combined and melted. Pour immediately over the top of the warm cake and let it drain down through the holes. Let cool.

4. Make the coconut cream by adding 2 cups of the cream portion of the coconut milk to a bowl. Beat with hand mixers on high for five minutes. Add in the Swerve sweetener and vanilla extract and mix until well combined. Once the cake has cooled completely, spread the coconut cream over the top and sprinkle with mini chocolate chips. Store in the fridge until ready to eat.

5. When ready to eat, make a batch of caramel sauce topping using ¼ cup of the Cashew Coconut Caramel Sauce and ¼ cup caramel chips with the same directions above in step number 3. Drizzle the warm caramel sauce over the cake and slice into 18 servings. Enjoy!

CASHEW COCONUT CARAMEL SAUCE
¾ cup salted cashews
¾ cup raw honey
½ cup softened coconut butter
2-3 Tbs. water
½ tsp. caramel or vanilla extract

1. Soak cashews in water for one hour. Drain and place in a high-powered blender with the rest of the ingredients and blend until smooth. Store in the fridge until ready to use.

2. When ready to use, place the caramel sauce in a saucepan over low heat and stir until warm and melted.

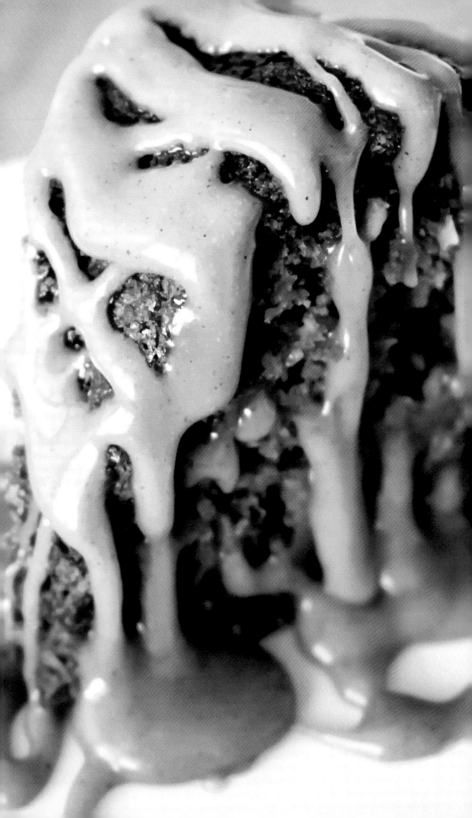

CARAMEL APPLE CAKE

Makes 16 servings
235 calories / 7.5F / 38C / 4P / per serving

1 cup raw honey
2 Tbs. grass-fed butter or coconut oil
2 Tbs. light tasting olive oil
2 large eggs
1 tsp. vanilla extract
4 cups peeled, shredded apples
2 cups white whole wheat flour
2 tsp. ground cinnamon
2 tsp. baking soda
2 tsp. ground nutmeg
1 tsp. sea salt
½ tsp. ground cloves

Caramel Sauce:
½ cup OffBeat Salted Caramel Butter, Cinnamon Bun Butter,
   or natural almond butter
½ cup raw honey
1 tsp. vanilla extract

1. Preheat oven to 350 degrees.

2. Beat the honey, butter and olive oil together in a bowl. Beat in the eggs and vanilla. Fold in the shredded apples then mix in all the dry ingredients.

3. Pour the batter into a well-greased Bundt pan. Bake for 45 minutes. Let cool for 30-60 minutes.

4. Make the Almond Caramel Sauce just before serving. In a small saucepan, mix the nut butter, honey and vanilla over medium heat. Stir constantly until all the ingredients melt together. Drizzle the caramel sauce evenly over the top of the cake. Slice into 16 servings. Enjoy!

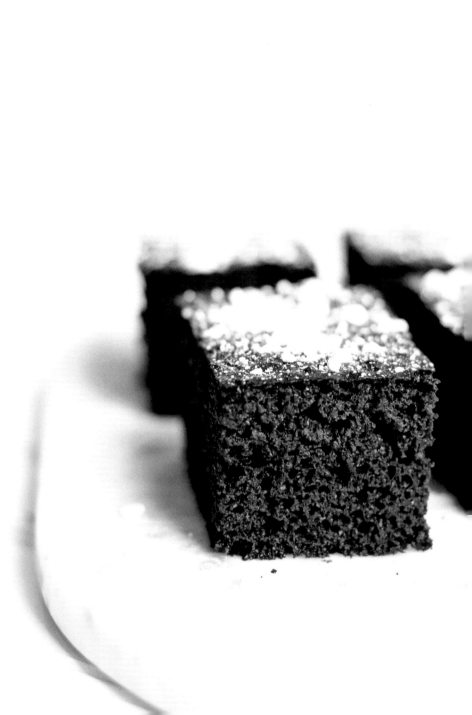

DEVIL'S FOOD CAKE

Makes 18 servings
165 calories / 6F / 22C / 5.5P / per serving

---

1 ½ cups fat-free milk
2 Tbs. lemon juice
28g Devil's Food (or chocolate) pudding mix
½ cup fat-free milk
½ cup grass-fed butter or coconut oil
1 cup coconut sugar
2 tsp. vanilla extract
1 large egg
4 egg whites
¼ cup unsweetened applesauce
1 ¾ cup white whole wheat flour
¾ cup cocoa powder
1 tsp. baking soda
1 tsp. baking powder
1 tsp. sea salt

1. Preheat the oven to 350 degrees.

2. Add 1 ½ cups milk and lemon juice to a small bowl; set aside. Combine the pudding mix with ½ cup milk in a bowl and whisk for 2 minutes. Store in the fridge until needed.

3. Beat the butter and coconut sugar together. Add the vanilla, egg, egg whites and applesauce. Mix until well combined; set aside.

4. In a large bowl, sift the flour, cocoa powder, baking soda, baking powder and sea salt. Stir until well combined. Add the dry ingredients to the wet ingredients and the milk/lemon juice mixture up over the top. Mix on low until just combined. Fold in the prepared pudding.

5. Pour the batter into a greased 9x13 pan. Bake for 30-35 minutes or until a toothpick comes out clean when inserted into the center. Slice into 18 servings. Enjoy!

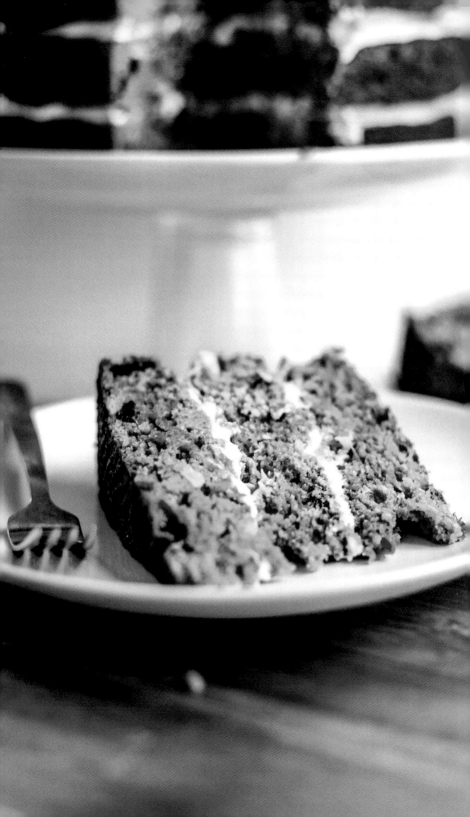

GOLDEN HONEY CARROT CAKE
Makes 20 servings
310 calories / 7.5F / 54C / 6P / per slice

6 cups grated carrots
1 cup coconut sugar
1 cup raisins
¼ cup grass-fed butter
2 large eggs
4 egg whites
1 Tbs. vanilla extract
1 cup raw honey
¾ cup unsweetened applesauce
1 cup crushed pineapple, drained
3 cups white whole wheat flour
1 Tbs. ground cinnamon
1 ½ tsp. baking soda
1 tsp. sea salt
½ cup chopped pecans
Frosting:
8 oz. Neufchâtel cream cheese
½ cup raw honey
2 Tbs. CSE Simply Vanilla Protein Powder

1. Preheat oven to 350.

2. Stir the grated carrots, coconut sugar and raisins together in a bowl; set aside.

3. Beat the butter in a large bowl until smooth. Add the egg, egg whites and vanilla; mix. Beat in the honey, applesauce and drained crushed pineapple last.

4. In a separate bowl, stir together the flour, cinnamon, baking soda and salt. Add to the wet mixture and stir until just combined. Fold in the carrot/raisin mixture and the pecans.

5. Grease three, 9 inch, round cake pans. Pour the batter evenly into each pan. Bake for 20-25 minutes. Let cool for 20 minutes in the pan, then remove and transfer to a cooling rack.

6. Beat all the frosting ingredients together. Once the cake is cooled, frost between each layer and stack. Use the remaining frosting to frost the top of the cake. Slice into 20 servings. Enjoy!

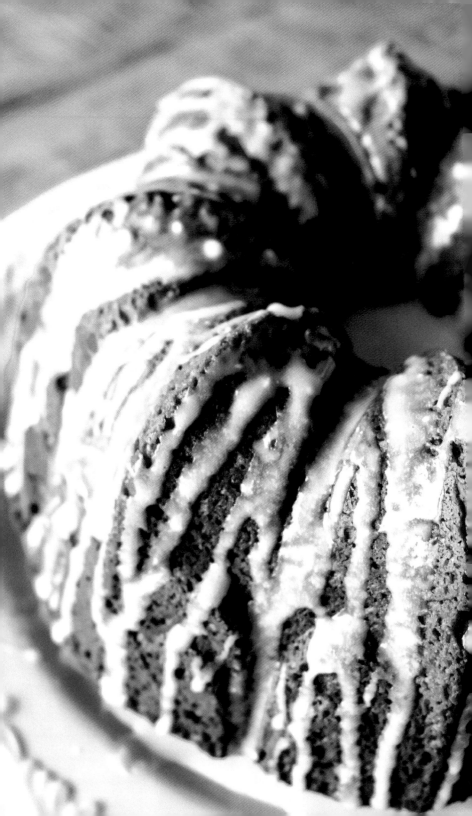

ICED VANILLA DONUT CAKE

Makes 16 servings
295 calories / 8.5F / 49C / 5P / per serving

---

3 cups white whole wheat flour
2 tsp. baking powder
½ tsp. baking soda
1 tsp. ground cinnamon
½ tsp. ground nutmeg
¼ tsp. sea salt
½ cup melted coconut oil
1 cup raw honey
½ cup pure maple syrup
½ cup unsweetened applesauce
2 cups mashed, cooked and peeled sweet potatoes
1 tsp. vanilla extract
4 large eggs
Vanilla Icing:
1 cup powdered sugar
2 Tbs. pasteurized egg whites
½ tsp. clear vanilla extract

1. Preheat oven to 350 degrees.

2. In a large bowl stir together the flour, baking powder, baking soda, cinnamon, nutmeg and sea salt; set aside.

3. In a separate bowl, beat together the melted coconut oil, honey, pure maple syrup and applesauce for three minutes. Add the mashed sweet potatoes and vanilla extract; mix well. Beat in one egg at a time. Then add the flour mixture and beat on low until just combined.

4. Pour the batter into a greased Bundt pan. Bake for 1 hour. Let cool 15-20 minutes in the pan and then tip over onto a serving plate and let cool before frosting.

5. In a large bowl, beat the powdered sugar, egg whites and vanilla extract together until well combined. Drizzle the icing evenly over the cooled cake. Let the icing harden before serving. Slice into 16 servings. Enjoy!

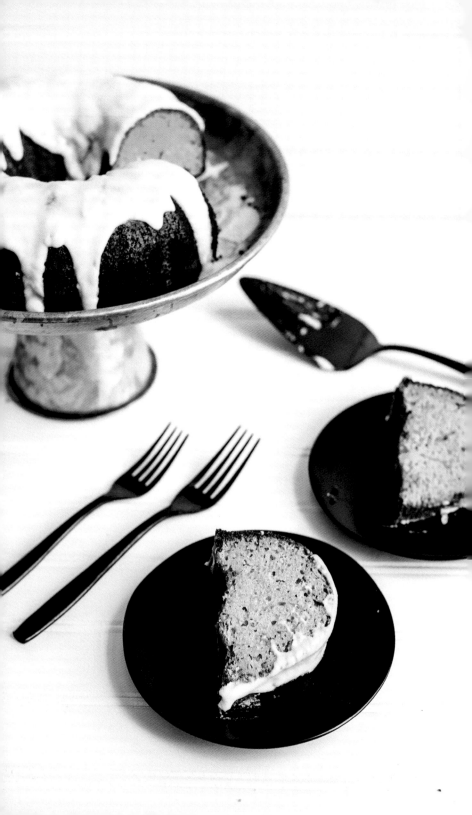

LEMON POUND CAKE

Makes 16 servings
315 calories / 7.5F / 57C / 5P / per slice

1 cup fat-free milk
2 Tbs. lemon juice
2 Tbs. lemon zest
½ cup grass-fed butter
1 ½ cups Swerve Confectioners Sweetener
¾ cup raw honey
3 large eggs
½ cup unsweetened applesauce
3 cups white whole wheat flour
½ tsp. baking soda
½ tsp. sea salt

Syrup:
⅓ cup water
⅓ cup Swerve sweetener
2 Tbs. lemon juice

Glaze:
1 cup powdered sugar
2 Tbs. pasteurized egg whites
1 Tbs. lemon juice
1 tsp. lemon zest
1 tsp. softened OffBeat Lemon Coconut Bliss Butter
     or coconut butter

1. Preheat oven to 325 degrees.

2. Place the milk, lemon juice and lemon zest in a small bowl; set aside.

3. Beat the butter, Swerve and honey together in a large bowl. Add in the eggs and applesauce; set aside.

4. In a separate bowl, combine the flour, baking soda and sea salt together. Add ½ of the dry mixture to the wet mixture, then add the milk and lemon juice mixture and then add the rest of the dry mixture on top. Mix until just combined.

5. Pour the batter into a greased Bundt pan. Bake for 60 minutes. Let cool for 10 minutes in the pan and then transfer to a cooling rack. Place a sheet of parchment paper under the cooling rack. Combine the syrup ingredients and then slowly pour over the cake while it's still warm. Let cool completely.

6. Beat the powdered sugar, egg whites, lemon juice, lemon zest and nut butter together in a large bowl until well combined. Drizzle icing evenly over the cooled cake. Let the icing harden before serving. Slice into 16 servings. Enjoy!

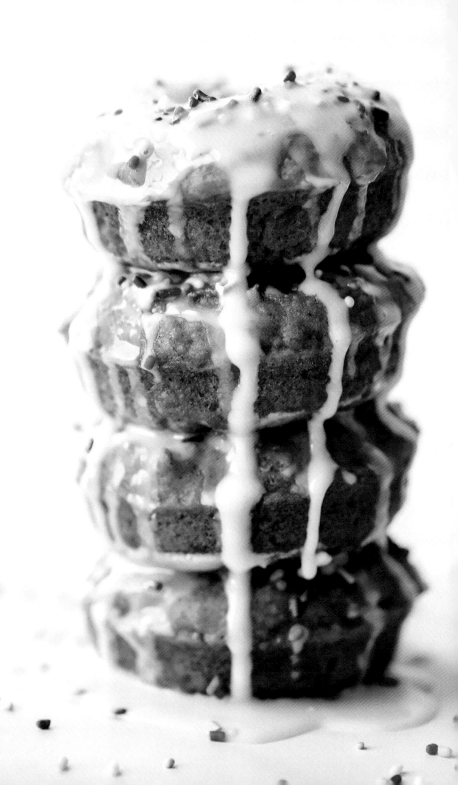

OLD-FASHIONED ICED CAKE DONUTS

Makes 12 servings
260 calories / 6F / 48C / 4P / per donut

1 ½ cups whole wheat pastry flour
1 tsp. baking powder
½ tsp. ground cinnamon
¼ tsp. baking soda
¼ tsp. ground nutmeg
1/8 tsp. sea salt
¼ cup melted coconut oil
½ cup raw honey
¼ cup pure maple syrup
¼ cup unsweetened applesauce
½ cup cooked, peeled & mashed sweet potatoes
½ tsp. vanilla extract
2 large eggs

Icing:
2 cups powdered sugar
4 Tbs. pasteurized egg whites
1 tsp. clear vanilla extract

Topping per donut:
½ tsp. candy sprinkles

1. Preheat oven to 350 degrees.

2. Combine all dry ingredients together in a large bowl; set aside.

3. In a separate bowl, beat the melted coconut oil, honey, pure maple syrup and applesauce for three minutes. Add the mashed sweet potatoes and vanilla extract; mix well. Beat in one egg at a time.

4. Add the dry ingredients to the wet ingredients and mix on low until well combined.

5. Spray a donut pan with cooking spray. Pour the mixture into a large piping bag or Ziploc bag. Cut a hole in the end of the bag and pipe the batter into the greased donut molds, making about 12 donuts. Bake for 13-15 minutes. Let cool in the pan for 2 minutes, then transfer to a cooling rack and let cool completely.

6. Beat the icing ingredients together in a large bowl until well combined. Place a piece of parchment paper under the cooling rack. Dip each donut into the icing, let the excess drip off into the bowl and then return to the cooling rack. Once the icing is firm, dip each donut a second time and immediately top with sprinkles. Enjoy!

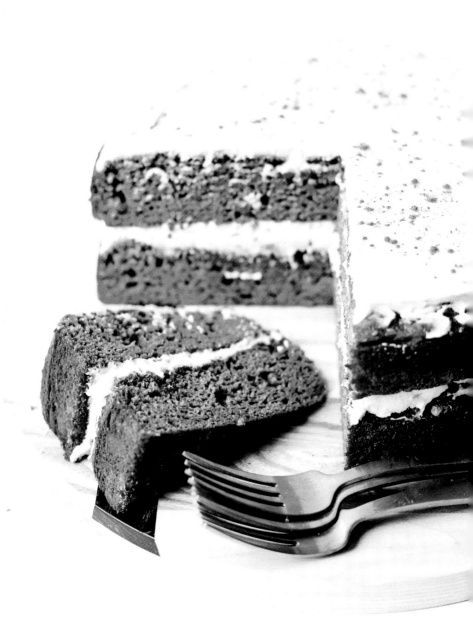

PUMPKIN CREAM CHEESE CAKE

Makes 16 servings
305 calories / 10F / 45C / 9P / per serving

2 ½ cups Kodiak Cakes Buttermilk Mix
1 serving CSE Simply Vanilla or Pumpkin Pie Protein Powder
1 tsp. ground cinnamon
1 tsp. ground cloves
1 tsp. ground nutmeg
1 tsp. pumpkin pie spice
1 tsp. sea salt
1 tsp. baking soda
2 ripe bananas
2 Tbs. grass-fed butter
½ cup raw honey
½ cup Swerve Confectioners Sweetener
2 cups canned pumpkin
4 large eggs

Crumble Topping:
¼ cup Kodiak Cakes Cinnamon Oat Mix
¼ cup coconut sugar
2 Tbs. grass-fed butter
1 tsp. ground cinnamon

Butter Cream Frosting:
6 oz. Neufchâtel cream cheese
¼ cup grass-fed butter
½ cup raw honey
1 tsp vanilla extract
Dash of cinnamon

1. Preheat oven to 350 degrees.

2. Combine all dry ingredients together in a large bowl; set aside.

3. In a large bowl, beat the bananas, butter, honey and Swerve together until smooth. Add the pumpkin and eggs. Mix until well combined. Add the dry ingredients to the bowl and mix well.

4. Grease two, 9-inch, round cake pans. Pour batter evenly into both pans. Combine the crumble topping ingredients together and sprinkle over the top of each cake. Bake for 25 minutes or until golden brown and cooked through. Let cool in the pan for 10-15 minutes, then transfer to a cooling rack.

5. Beat the frosting ingredients together. Spread in between the two cake rounds and on the top. Slice into 16 servings. Enjoy! Store extras in the fridge.

PUMPKIN SHEET CAKE

Makes 15 servings
205 calories / 6F / 35C / 3P / per serving

1 cup white whole wheat flour
½ tsp baking powder
½ tsp baking soda
½ tsp sea salt
¼ tsp ground cinnamon
Dash of ground nutmeg
1 cup canned pumpkin
1 cup raw honey
2 large eggs
2 Tbs. melted coconut oil
2 tsp. vanilla extract

Frosting:
8 oz. Neufchâtel cream cheese
½ cup raw honey
1 tsp vanilla extract

1. Preheat oven to 350 degrees.

2. In a medium sized bowl, mix the flour, baking powder, baking soda, sea salt, cinnamon and nutmeg; set aside.

3. In a separate bowl, beat together the pumpkin, honey, eggs, melted coconut oil and vanilla. Add the wet ingredients to the dry ingredients and mix until just combined.

4. Pour the batter into a greased 9x13 baking dish and bake for 25 minutes. Let cool.

5. While the cake is baking, beat together the frosting ingredients. Store in the fridge until ready to use.

6. Frost the cake once cooled. Slice into 15 servings and Enjoy! Store extras in the fridge.

PSIDE DOWN PUMPKIN PIE

Makes 16 slices
230 calories / 11.5F / 27C / 5P / per slice

2 large eggs
1 cup unsweetened almond milk
2 cups canned pumpkin
½ cup raw honey
½ serving CSE Simply Vanilla or Pumpkin Pie Protein Powder
1 tsp. ground cinnamon
2 tsp. pumpkin pie spice

Crust:
⅔ cup almonds
⅔ cup cashews
⅔ cup unsweetened shredded coconut
⅔ cup old-fashioned rolled oats
¼ cup flaxseed meal
1 Tbs. vanilla extract
½ tsp. sea salt
20 dates, pitted

Topping per serving:
2 Tbs. spray whipped cream

1. Preheat oven to 425 degrees.

2. Place the eggs in blender and blend until frothy. Add the milk, pumpkin, honey, protein powder, cinnamon and pumpkin pie spice to the blender. Blend on low for 2 minutes.

3. Spray two, 9-inch pie rounds with cooking spray or line with a round piece of parchment paper. Pour half of the mixture into each round and bake for 15 minutes. Turn the heat down to 350 degrees and bake an additional 40 minutes. Refrigerate for at least two hours.

4. Make the crust topping by placing the almonds and cashews into a high-powered blender; pulse until broken up. Pour into a bowl, then add the shredded coconut, rolled oats, flaxseed meal, vanilla and sea salt to the bowl. Add the pitted dates to the blender and pulse until it turns into a paste. Add it to the bowl and mix well.

5. Once the pie is cooled, spread half of the crust mixture over each pie. Slice into 16 servings and top each serving with spray whipped cream. Enjoy!

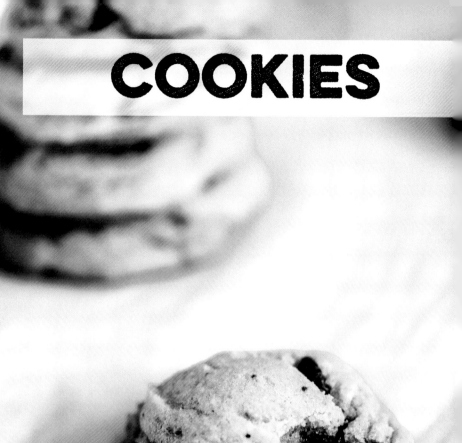

COOKIES

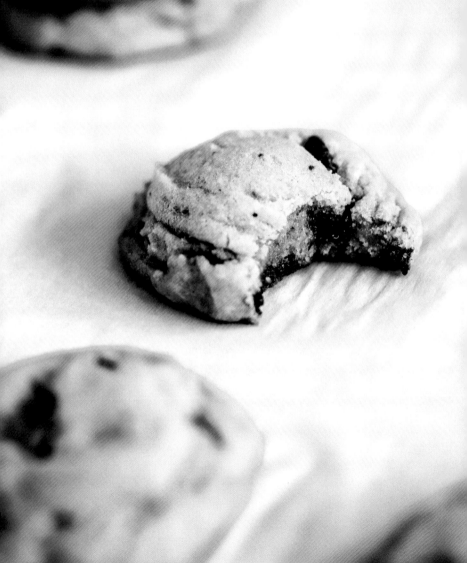

IT'S HARD TO BE SAD WHEN YOU'RE EATING A COOKIE

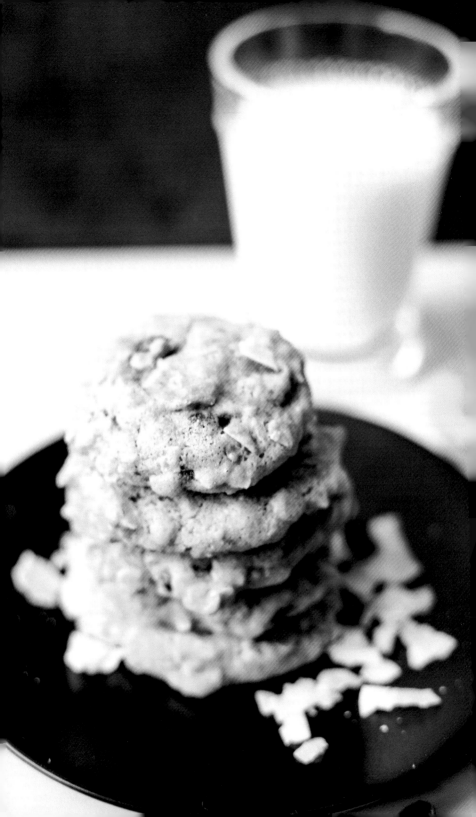

ALMOND JOY COOKIES

Makes 30 cookies
110 calories / 4.5F / 15.5C / 2.5P / per cookie

¼ cup OffBeat Midnight Almond Coconut Butter, Aloha Butter,
   or natural almond butter
¼ cup softened coconut butter
¾ cup raw honey
2 large eggs
½ tsp. almond extract
½ tsp. coconut extract
1 ½ cups white whole wheat flour
1 cup old-fashioned rolled oats
1 tsp. baking soda
½ tsp. sea salt
½ cup dark chocolate chips
½ cup unsweetened, flaked coconut
¼ cup chopped almonds

1. Preheat oven to 375 degrees.

2. Mix the nut butter, coconut butter and honey together in a bowl.
Beat in the eggs and extracts; set aside.

3. In a separate bowl, combine the flour, rolled oats, baking soda
and sea salt. Add the dry ingredients to the wet ingredients and mix
until just combined. Fold in the chocolate chips, flaked coconut and
chopped almonds.

4. Using a small cookie scoop, scoop onto a baking sheet lined with
parchment paper (makes 30 cookies). Bake for 7 minutes. Let cool on
the cookie sheet for 2 minutes, then transfer to a cooling rack. Enjoy!

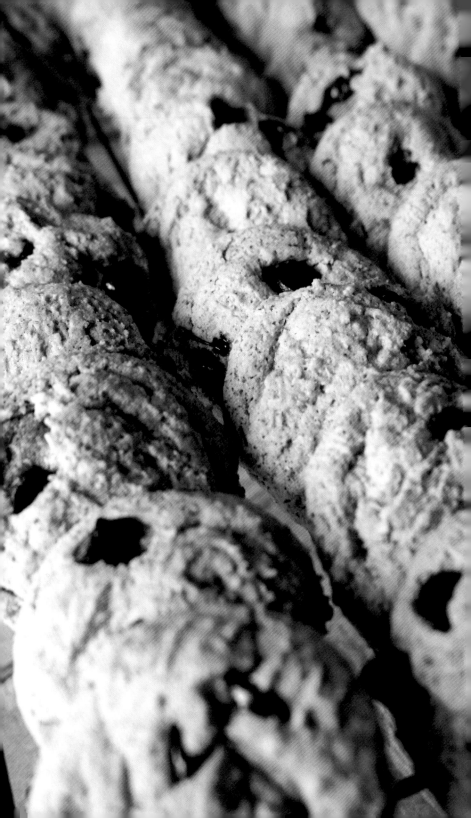

CAVEMAN COOKIES

Makes 22 cookies
120 calories / 7F / 11.5C / 3.5P / per cookie

1 ½ cups almond flour
¾ cup OffBeat Sweet Classic Peanut Butter, Candy Bar Butter,
    or natural peanut butter
½ cup raw honey
1 large egg
1 serving CSE Simply Vanilla Protein Powder
1 tsp. vanilla extract
1 tsp. baking soda
½ tsp. sea salt
½ cup dark chocolate chips

1. Preheat oven to 350 degrees.

2. Mix all the ingredients together, stirring in the chocolate chips last. Batter will be thick and sticky.

3. Using a small cookie scoop, scoop dough into balls and place on a baking sheet lined with parchment paper (makes 22 cookies). Bake for 7 minutes. Let cool for 2 minutes, then transfer to a cooling rack. Enjoy!

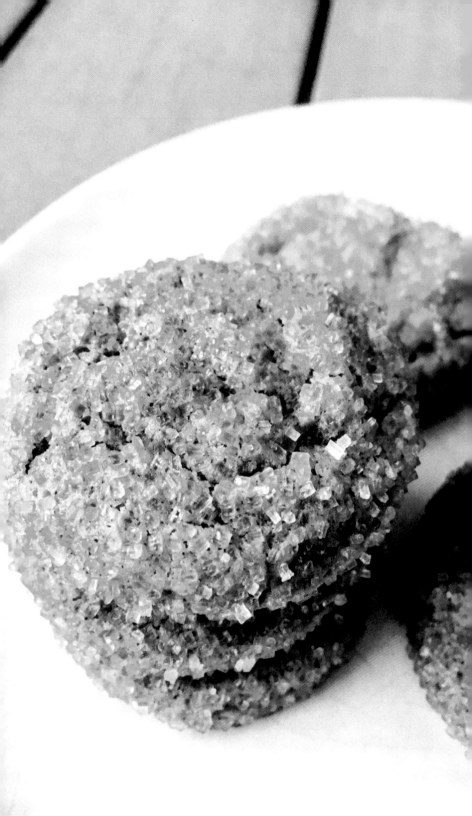

CHEWY GINGERSNAP COOKIES

Makes 34 cookies
110 calories / 4F / 17C / 2P / per cookie

¼ cup OffBeat Gingerbread Cookie Butter, Cinnamon Bun Butter,
    or natural almond butter
½ cup coconut oil or grass-fed butter
1 large egg
1 tsp. vanilla extract
¾ cup raw honey
⅓ cup molasses
2 ½ cups white whole wheat flour
1 tsp. baking soda
½ tsp. sea salt
½ tsp. ground cloves
2 tsp. ground ginger
2 tsp. ground cinnamon
½ cup organic sugar in the raw

1. Beat the nut butter and coconut oil/butter together. Add the egg and vanilla. Slowly beat in the honey and molasses; set aside.

2. In a separate bowl, mix the flour, baking soda, salt, cloves, ginger and cinnamon. Add the dry ingredients to the wet ingredients and mix until just combined. Cover and chill in the fridge for one hour.

3. Preheat oven to 350 degrees.

4. Remove the dough from the fridge. Using a small cookie scoop, drop round balls of dough into the raw sugar one at a time. Roll around until well-coated. Place on a baking sheet lined with parchment paper (makes 34 cookies). Bake for 8-10 minutes. Let cool for 2 minutes, then transfer to a cooling rack. Enjoy!

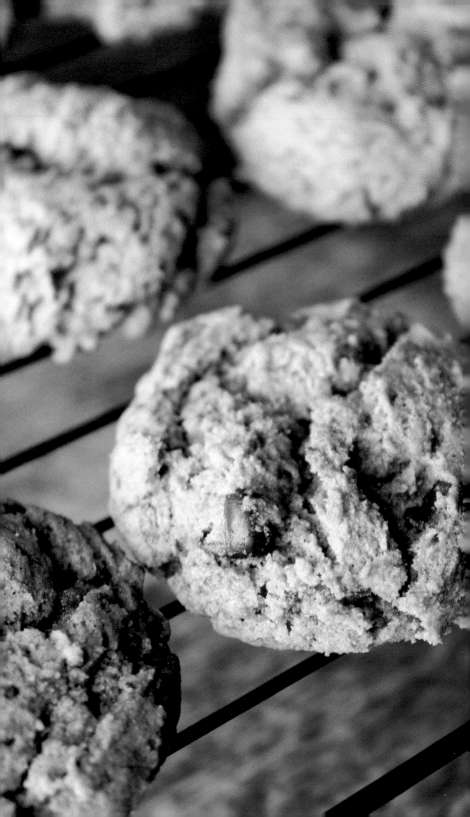

CLASSIC CHOCOLATE CHIPPERS

Makes 42 cookies
100 calories / 5.5F / 11C / 1.5P / per cookie

---

1 cup coconut oil or grass-fed butter, softened
¾ cup coconut sugar
½ cup xylitol sweetener
2 large eggs
1 Tbs. vanilla extract
2 ¾ cup white whole wheat flour
1 tsp. baking soda
1 tsp. sea salt
½ cup dark chocolate chips

1. Preheat oven to 375 degrees.

2. Beat coconut oil/butter, coconut sugar and xylitol in a bowl until smooth. Add the eggs and vanilla until just combined.

3. Sprinkle in 2 cups of flour, baking soda, sea salt and chocolate chips. Top with remaining ¾ cups of flour. Mix on low until all ingredients are incorporated.

4. Using a small cookie scoop, scoop cookie dough onto a baking sheet lined with parchment paper (makes 42 cookies). Bake for 8-9 minutes. Let cool for 2 minutes, then transfer to a cooling rack. Enjoy!

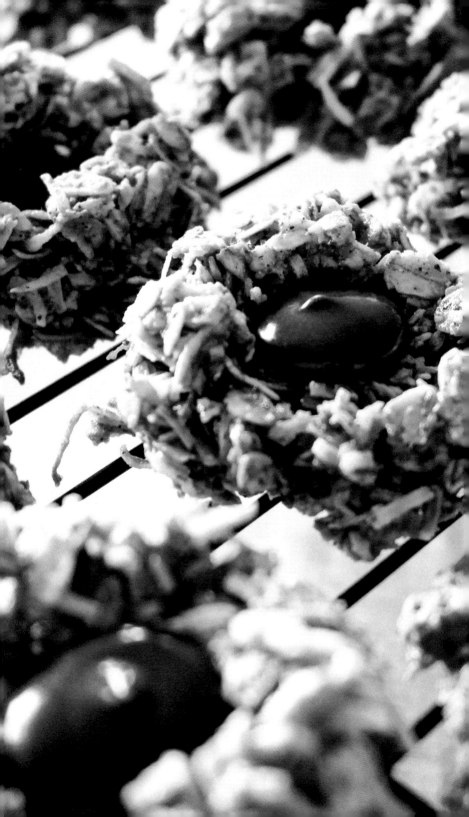

COCONOAT MACAROONS

Makes 22 cookies
135 calories / 9F / 14C / 2P / per cookie

¼ cup melted coconut oil
¼ cup OffBeat Aloha Butter, Midnight Almond Coconut Butter, or natural almond butter
1 large egg
½ cup coconut sugar
2 cups old-fashioned rolled oats
1 cup unsweetened shredded coconut
Dash sea salt
Dash ground cinnamon
22 large chocolate chunks or Cadbury Mini Eggs (great for Easter)

1. Preheat oven to 325 degrees.

2. Beat the coconut oil, nut butter, egg and coconut sugar together until smooth. Add the oats, shredded coconut, sea salt and cinnamon. Mix until well combined.

3. Scoop rounded tablespoons of dough onto a baking sheet lined with parchment paper (makes 22 cookies). Bake for 8 minutes. Remove from the oven and press a chocolate chunk or Cadbury Egg in the middle of each macaroon. Let cool for 5 minutes and then transfer to a cooling rack. Enjoy!

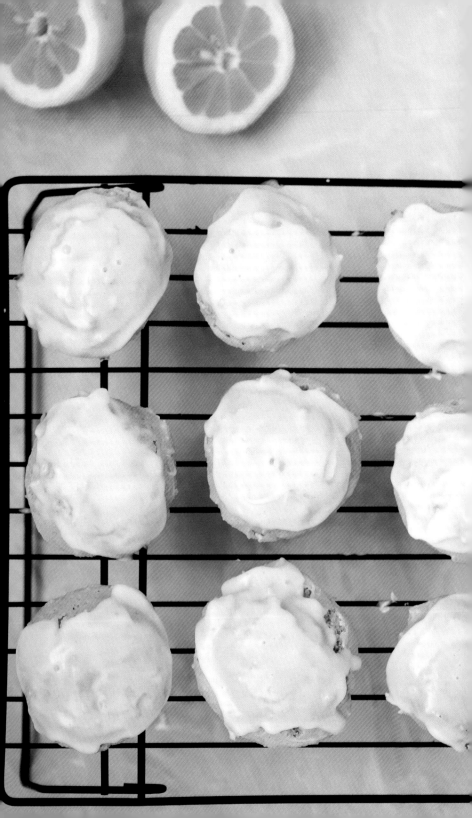

LEMON DROP COOKIES

Makes 16 cookies
140 calories / 6F / 18.5C / 3.5P / per cookie

---

1 large egg
¼ cup unsweetened almond milk
¼ cup raw honey or pure maple syrup
2 Tbs. melted coconut oil
1 Tbs. lemon juice
2 tsp. lemon extract
1 cup whole wheat pastry flour
1 cup almond flour
½ serving CSE Simply Vanilla Protein Powder
1 tsp. baking powder
½ tsp. sea salt
1 Tbs. lemon zest
Icing:
1 cup powdered sugar
2 Tbs. pasteurized egg whites

1. Preheat oven to 375 degrees.

2. In a large bowl beat the egg, almond milk, honey/syrup, melted coconut oil, lemon juice and lemon extract together; set aside.

3. In a separate bowl, stir together the flours, protein powder, baking powder and sea salt. Add the wet ingredients to the dry ingredients and mix until well combined. Fold in the lemon zest.

4. Using a small cookie scoop, scoop the dough into balls and place on a cookie sheet lined with parchment paper (makes 16 cookies). Bake for 5-6 minutes or until lightly golden on the bottom. Transfer to a cooling rack.

5. Beat together the powdered sugar and egg whites. Once the cookies are cooled off, place a sheet of parchment or wax paper underneath the cooling rack and drizzle each cookie with the icing. Enjoy!

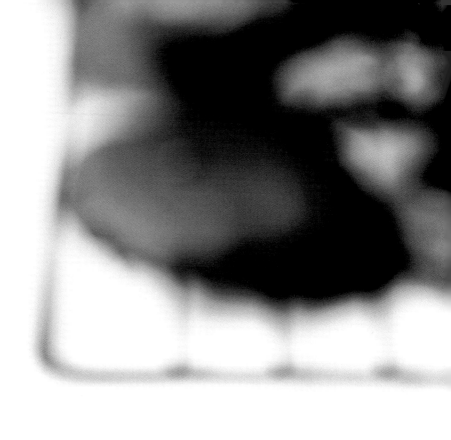
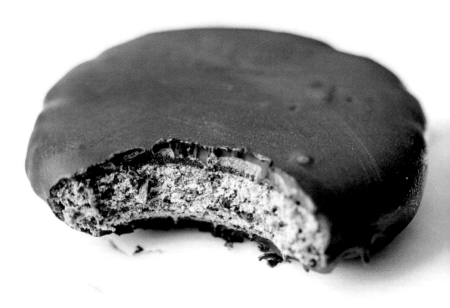

MINT CHOCOLATE COOKIES

Makes 36 cookies
150 calories / 7.5F / 17C / 4P / per cookie

---

12 oz. OffBeat Mint Chocolate Chip Cookie Butter
½ cup raw honey
2 servings CSE Brownie Batter or Mint Chocolate Cookie Protein
    Powder
1 cup Kodiak Cakes Buttermilk Mix
½ tsp. vanilla extract
Pinch of sea salt
2 cups dark chocolate chips
1 Tbs. coconut oil

1. Add the OffBeat Butter, honey, protein powder, Kodiak Cakes Mix, vanilla and salt together in a bowl. Mix until well combined. Using a small cookie scoop, scoop them onto a baking sheet lined with parchment paper (makes 36 cookies). Using the bottom of a glass jar or cup, smash the balls flat and then round out the edges with your hands to form into a cookie. Place the cookies in the freezer for 30 minutes or until hardened.

2. Place the dark chocolate and coconut oil into a small saucepan over low heat to melt (or melt in a bowl in the microwave). Stir continuously until completely melted, then turn the heat off. Drop each cookie into the chocolate one at a time and scoop them out with a fork, letting the excess chocolate drip off into the pan. Place the chocolate dipped cookies back onto the parchment paper and then place them in the freezer to harden.

3. Once frozen, transfer to a storage container or bag. When ready to eat, let cookies sit out 5-10 minutes to thaw before taking a bite. Enjoy!

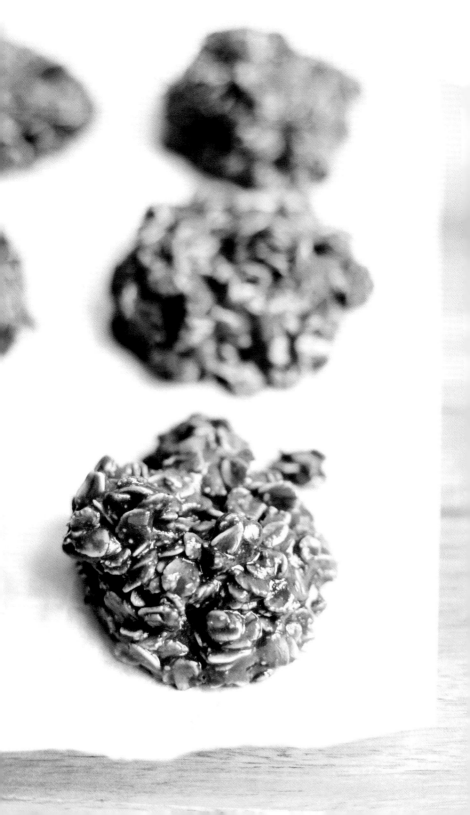

NO-BAKE COOKIES

Makes 8 cookies
280 calories / 15.5F / 29.5C / 6P / per cookie

¼ cup unsweetened almond milk
⅓ cup xylitol sweetener
⅓ cup raw honey
2 Tbs. cocoa powder
¼ cup grass-fed butter or coconut oil
½ cup OffBeat Sweet Classic Peanut Butter,
    Buckeye Brownie Peanut Butter, or natural peanut butter
Dash of sea salt
1 ½ cups old-fashioned rolled oats

1. Whisk the almond milk, xylitol, honey, cocoa powder and coconut oil or butter together in a saucepan. Bring to a boil and stir for one minute. Turn heat down to low.

2. Stir in the peanut butter, sea salt and oats until well combined. Remove from the heat.

3. Spoon ¼ cup of the mixture onto a cookie sheet lined with parchment paper to make one cookie. Continue with the rest of the mixture (makes 8 cookies). Let set in the fridge for 30-60 minutes. Enjoy!

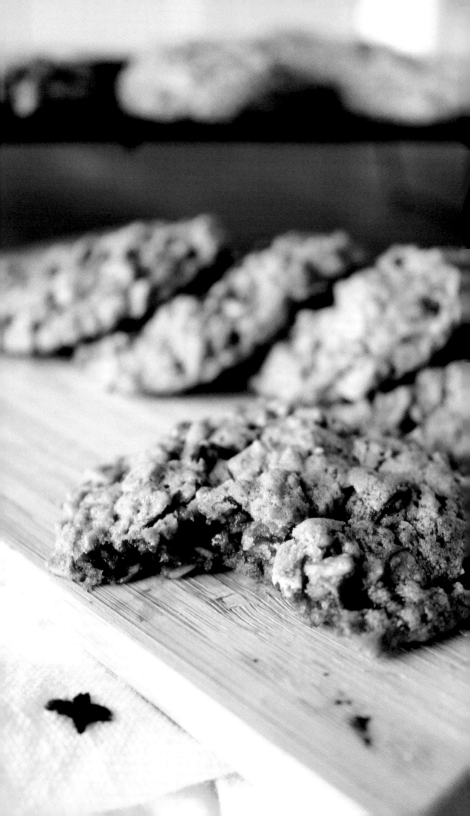

OATMEAL PB CHOCOLATE CHIP COOKIES
Makes 20 cookies
140 calories / 9F / 12C / 3.5P / per cookie

½ cup grass-fed butter or softened coconut oil
⅓ cup coconut sugar
1 serving CSE Simply Vanilla Protein Powder
¼ cup OffBeat Sweet Classic Peanut Butter
    or natural peanut butter
2 large eggs
1 tsp. vanilla extract
2 cups old-fashioned rolled oats
1 tsp. baking soda
Dash of sea salt
½ cup extra dark chocolate chips

1. Preheat oven to 375 degrees.

2. Mix the butter, coconut sugar, protein powder and the peanut butter together in a bowl. Add the eggs and vanilla; mix until smooth.

3. In a separate bowl, combine the oats, baking soda and salt. Add the dry ingredients to the wet ingredients and mix until just combined. Stir in the chocolate chips last.

4. Using a small cookie scoop, scoop the cookie dough onto a baking sheet lined with parchment paper (makes 20 cookies). Bake for 6-7 minutes. Let cool 2 minutes, then transfer to a cooling rack. Enjoy!

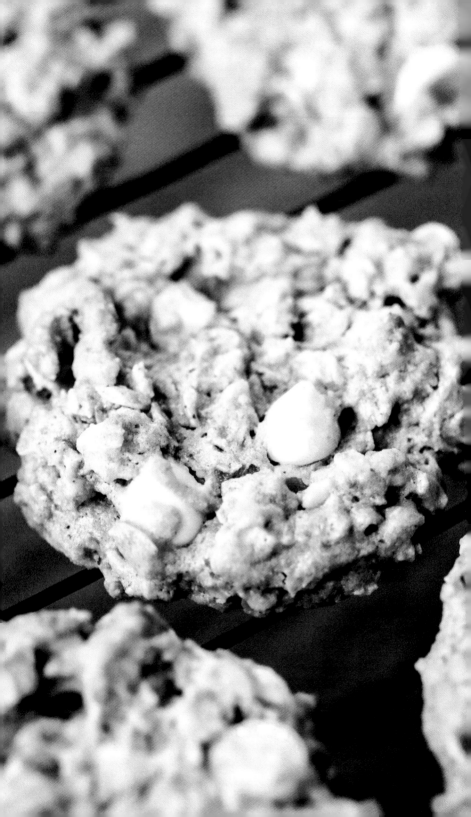

PEANUT BUTTER BLONDIE COOKIES

Makes 24 cookies
120 calories / 5.5F / 14C / 4P / per cookie

1 cup OffBeat Sweet Classic Peanut Butter
    or natural peanut butter
½ cup raw honey
2 Tbs. grass-fed butter
1 large egg
1 tsp. vanilla extract
2 cups old-fashioned rolled oats
1 serving CSE Simply Vanilla Protein Powder
½ tsp. baking soda
¼ tsp. sea salt
½ cup vanilla milk chocolate or white chocolate chips

1. Preheat oven to 350 degrees.

2. Beat the peanut butter, honey and butter together in a bowl. Beat in the egg and vanilla extract; set aside.

3. In a separate bowl, add the oats, protein powder, baking soda and sea salt and mix. Add the wet ingredients to the dry ingredients and mix until just combined. Fold in the chocolate chips.

4. Using a small cookie scoop, scoop dough onto a baking sheet lined with parchment paper (makes 24 cookies). Bake for 8-10 minutes. Let cool 2 minutes, then transfer to a cooling rack. Enjoy!

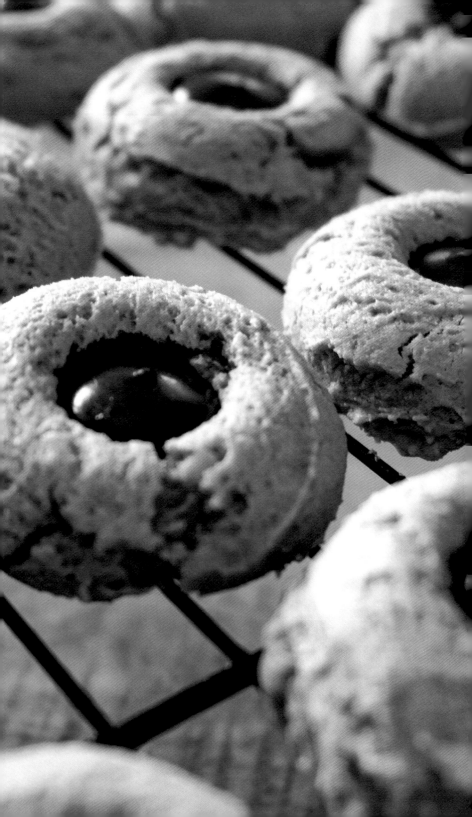

PEANUT BUTTER KISS COOKIES

Makes 24 cookies
125 calories / 6F / 13C / 5P / per cookie

½ cup OffBeat Sweet Classic Peanut Butter
   or natural peanut butter
½ cup raw honey
2 Tbs. melted coconut oil
2 large eggs
1 tsp. vanilla extract
1 ½ cup Kodiak Cakes Buttermilk Mix
1 serving CSE Simply Vanilla Protein Powder
1 tsp. baking soda
1 tsp. baking powder
¼ tsp. sea salt
24 Hershey's chocolate kisses
   or Guittard super cookie chocolate chips

1. Preheat oven to 350 degrees.

2. Beat the peanut butter, honey and coconut oil together in a bowl. Beat in the eggs and vanilla extract; set aside.

3. In a separate bowl, add the Kodiak Cakes Mix, protein powder, baking soda, baking powder and sea salt; mix well. Add the dry ingredients to the wet ingredients and mix on low until just combined.

4. Using a small cookie scoop, scoop dough onto a baking sheet lined with parchment paper (makes 24 cookies). Bake for 5 minutes. Unwrap the chocolate kisses and place one in the center of each cookie. Transfer to a cooling rack. Enjoy!

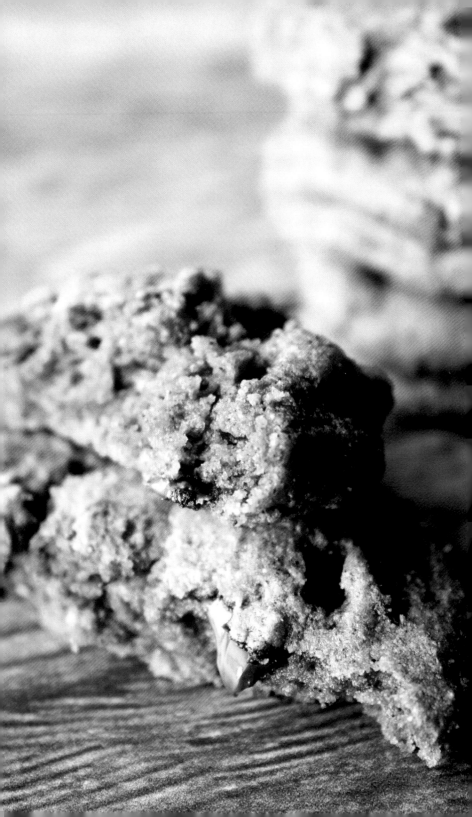

PUMPKIN CHOCOLATE CHIP COOKIES

Makes 24 cookies
170 calories / 7F / 24C / 4P / per cookie

1 cup coconut sugar
½ cup grass-fed butter, softened
1 cup canned pumpkin
1 large egg
1 Tbs. vanilla extract
3 cups Kodiak Cakes Buttermilk Mix
1 tsp. baking powder
1 tsp. baking soda
2 tsp. ground cinnamon
½ tsp. ground cloves
½ tsp. ground nutmeg
¼ tsp. sea salt
1 cup dark chocolate chips

1. Preheat oven to 350 degrees.

2. Beat together the coconut sugar and butter. Add the pumpkin, egg and vanilla. Mix well and set aside.

3. In a separate bowl, combine the Kodiak Cakes Mix, baking powder, baking soda, spices and sea salt. Add the wet ingredients to the dry ingredients and stir until just combined. Fold in the chocolate chips.

4. Using a large cookie scoop, drop dough onto a baking sheet lined with parchment paper (makes 24 cookies). Bake for 10-12 minutes. Let cool 2 minutes and then transfer to a cooling rack. Enjoy!

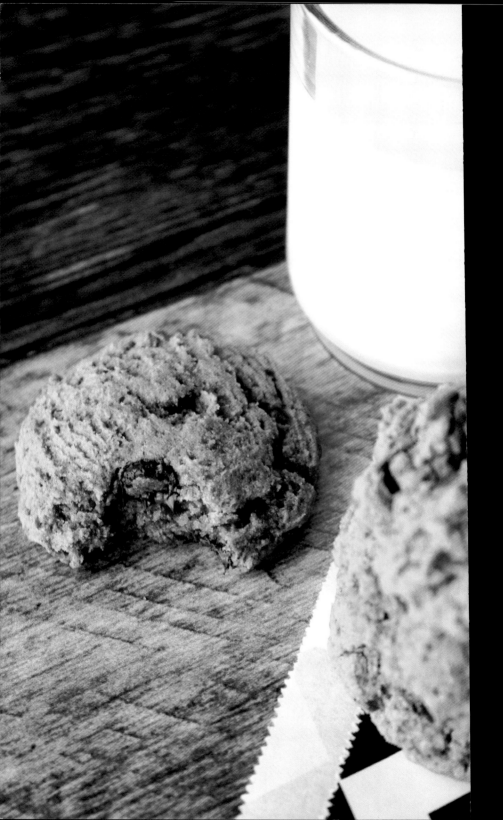

PUMPKIN SPICE COOKIES

Makes 26 cookies
140 calories / 5F / 20C / 3P / per cookie

½ cup grass-fed butter
1 cup coconut sugar
¼ cup raw honey
1 tsp. vanilla extract
1 large egg
⅓ cup canned pumpkin
½ tsp. baking soda
1 tsp. ground cinnamon
¼ tsp. ground ginger
¼ tsp. sea salt
⅛ tsp. ground cloves
⅛ tsp. ground nutmeg
2 ½ cups Kodiak Cakes Buttermilk Mix
½ cup dark chocolate chips

1. Preheat oven to 350 degrees.

2. Beat the butter, coconut sugar and honey together in a large bowl. Add the vanilla, egg and pumpkin. Beat until well combined; set aside.

3. In a separate bowl, combine all the dry ingredients. Add the wet ingredients to the dry ingredients and stir until well combined. Fold in the chocolate chips.

4. Using a small cookie scoop, scoop into balls and place on a baking sheet lined with parchment paper (makes 26 cookies). Bake for 10-12 minutes. Let cool 2 minutes, then transfer to a cooling rack. Enjoy!

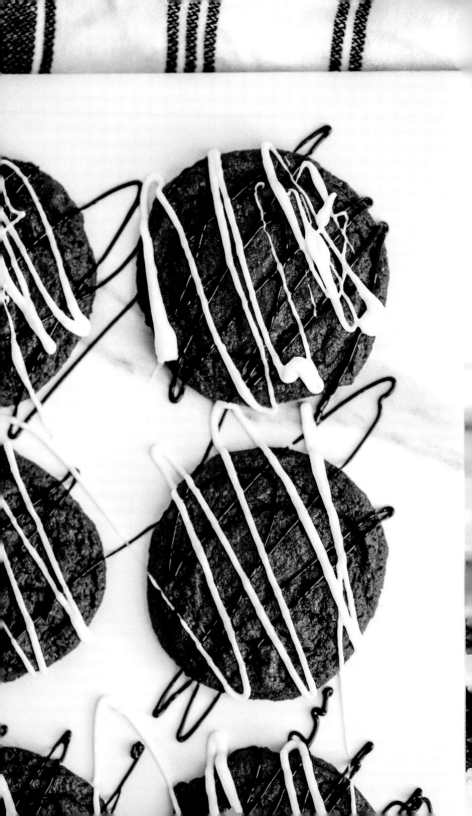

ED VELVET COOKIES

Makes 26 cookies
115 calories / 5F / 15C / 2.5P / per cookie

½ cup grass-fed butter or coconut oil
¾ cup raw honey
1 large egg
1 tsp. vanilla extract
2 cups Kodiak Cakes Buttermilk Mix
2 Tbs. beet root powder
1 serving CSE Simply Vanilla, Brownie Batter,
   or Strawberry Cheesecake Protein Powder
2 Tbs. cocoa powder
1 tsp. baking powder
¼ tsp. sea salt

Chocolate Drizzle Topping:
30 dark chocolate chips, melted
30 white chocolate chips, melted

1. Beat butter/coconut oil and honey together until well combined.
Beat in the egg and vanilla; set aside.

2. In a separate bowl, combine the Kodiak Cakes Mix, beet root
powder, protein powder, cocoa powder, baking powder and sea
salt. Add the dry ingredients to the wet ingredients and mix until just
combined. Let cool in the fridge for 1 hour.

3. Preheat the oven to 350 degrees. Using a small cookie scoop,
scoop the sticky dough balls onto a baking sheet lined with parchment paper (makes 26 cookies). Bake for 8-10 minutes or until lightly
browned on top.

4. Let cool for 2 minutes and then transfer to a cooling rack. Add
the white and dark chocolate chips to two separate bowls. Melt in
the microwave for 30 seconds at a time until they are melted and
smooth, stirring in between. Drizzle the dark chocolate over each
cookie, then repeat with the white chocolate. Allow the chocolate to
harden. Enjoy!

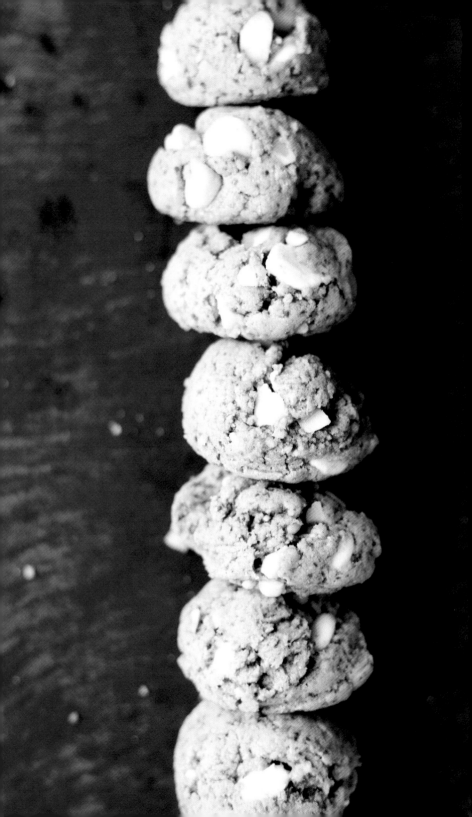

WHITE CHOCOLATE MACADAMIA COOKIES

Makes 24 cookies
125 calories / 7.5F / 11.5C / 3.5P / per cookie

½ cup coconut oil or grass-fed butter, softened
½ cup coconut sugar
1 serving CSE Simply Vanilla Protein Powder
1 large egg
1 tsp. vanilla extract
1½ cups white whole wheat flour
1 tsp. baking soda
½ tsp. sea salt
½ cup white chocolate chips
½ cup chopped macadamia nuts

1. Preheat oven to 350 degrees.

2. Beat coconut oil or butter together with the coconut sugar and protein powder. Beat in the egg and vanilla; set aside.

3. In a separate bowl, stir the flour, baking soda and sea salt together. Add the dry mixture to the wet mixture; mix well. Fold in the macadamia nuts and white chocolate chips.

4. Using a small cookie scoop, scoop the cookie dough on a baking sheet lined with parchment paper (makes 24 cookies). Bake for 8 minutes. Let cool for 2 minutes, then transfer to a cooling rack. Enjoy!

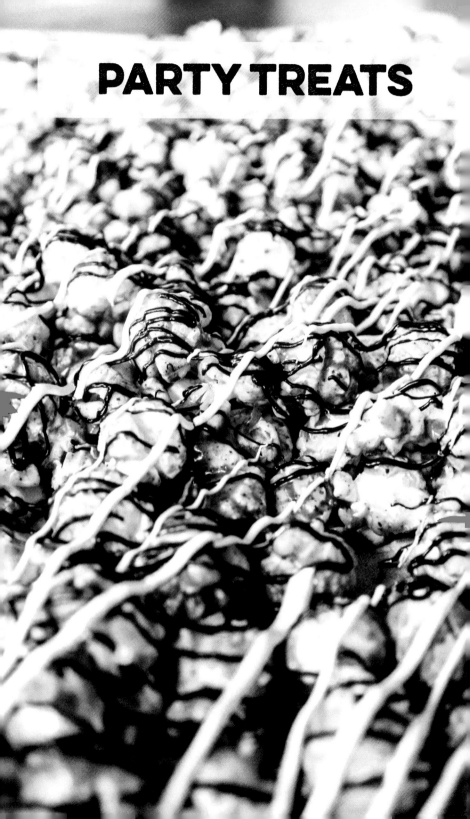

PARTY TREATS

GOOD FOOD IS ALL THE SWEETER WHEN SHARED WITH GOOD FRIENDS

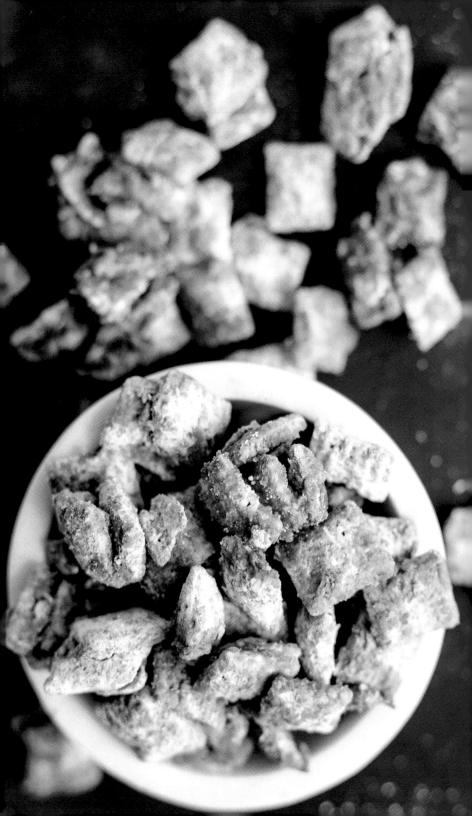

BROWNIE BATTER BUDDIES
Makes 16 servings / ½ cup (45g) per serving
185 calories / 5F / 29C / 7P / per serving

¾ cup raw honey
½ cup OffBeat Sweet Classic Peanut Butter,
    Buckeye Brownie Peanut Butter, or natural peanut butter
1 tsp. vanilla extract
1 serving CSE Brownie Batter
    or Chocolate Peanut Butter Protein Powder
1 Tbs. cocoa powder
3 cups Rice Chex cereal
1 cup powdered peanut butter

1. In a small saucepan melt together the honey, peanut butter and vanilla over low heat. Stir until melted together and smooth then remove from heat. Stir in the protein powder and cocoa powder.

2. Place Chex cereal into a large bowl. Pour the hot mixture over the top and gently stir until the cereal is well-coated.

3. Pour the chocolate Chex mixture into a large Ziploc bag, then dump the powdered peanut butter over the top. Seal the bag and shake until the cereal is well-coated. Pour out onto wax or parchment paper to cool. Store leftovers in the fridge. Enjoy!

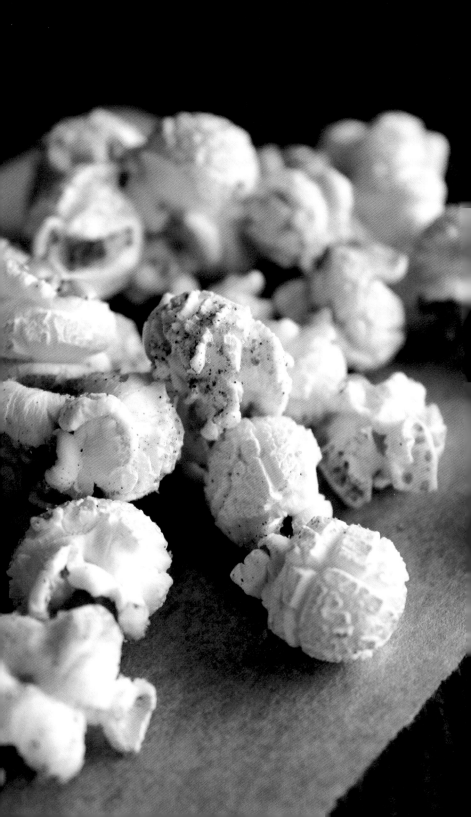

CHURRO POPCORN
Makes 1 serving
140 calories / 1F / 31C / 3P

3 cups (2 Tbs. kernels) air-popped popcorn
Coconut oil cooking spray
1 Tbs. brown sugar or coconut sugar
Pinch of sea salt
Dash of cinnamon

1. Use an air popper to pop the kernels, then dump out onto a sheet of parchment paper. Spray the tops well with cooking spray, then dump into a large Ziploc bag.

2. Add salt, sugar and cinnamon to the bag and shake until well coated. Enjoy!

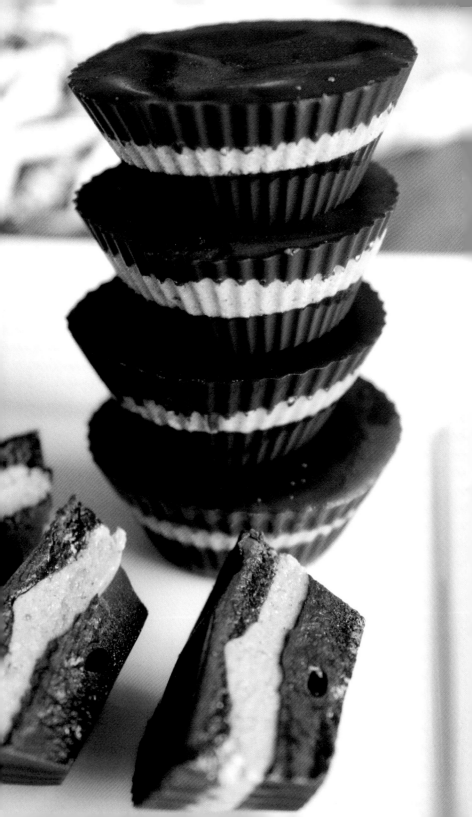

DARK CHOCOLATE PEANUT BUTTER CUPS

Makes 16 servings
130 calories / 9.5F / 8C / 3P / per peanut butter cup

1/2 cup coconut oil
1/4 cup raw honey
1/2 cup cocoa powder
1/4 cup OffBeat Sweet Classic Peanut Butter, Candy Bar Butter,
   or natural peanut butter
1/4 cup powdered peanut butter
1/2 serving CSE Simply Vanilla Protein Powder
1 Tbs. raw honey
1/2 tsp. vanilla extract
Pinch of sea salt
16 mini silicone baking cups

1. Melt the coconut oil, honey and cocoa powder together in a saucepan over low/medium heat. Whisk until well combined. Remove from heat.

2. Place 1/2 tablespoon of the chocolate mixture into each mini baking cup. Then place in the freezer to harden for 30 minutes.

3. Combine the peanut butter, powdered peanut butter, protein powder, honey, vanilla and sea salt in a bowl; set aside.

4. Once the chocolate is hardened, add a rounded teaspoon of the peanut butter filling to each mini baking cup. Press down to flatten the filling and fully cover the chocolate. Then pour another 1/2 tablespoon of the chocolate mixture over the peanut butter filling. Return the peanut butter cups to the freezer for at least 60 minutes.

5. To store the leftovers, pop out each peanut butter cup and place them in a freezer bag and store in the freezer. Let sit out for 5-10 minutes to soften before eating. Enjoy!

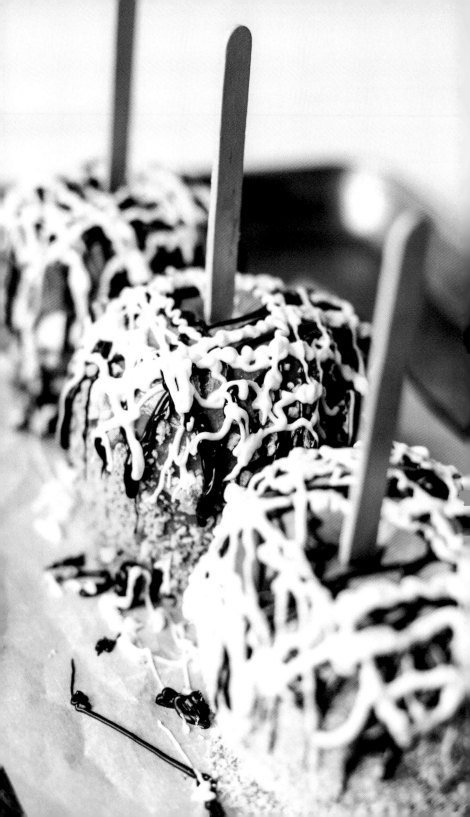

GOURMET CARAMEL APPLES

Makes 8 servings
285 calories / 10.5F / 44C / 4P / per apple w/o optional toppings

3 medium-sized apples
3 popsicle sticks
1/2 cup OffBeat Salted Caramel Butter, Sweet Classic Peanut Butter,
    Candy Bar Butter, Cinnamon Bun Butter, or natural almond butter
1/2 cup raw honey
1/2 tsp. vanilla extract

Toppings:
2 Tbs. (30 pieces) dark chocolate chips
2 Tbs. (30 pieces) white chocolate chips

Optional toppings:
Chopped nuts
Unsweetened shredded coconut
Mini chocolate chips
Chopped pretzels
Graham cracker crumbs

1. Wash apples, pat dry and remove stems. Pierce apples down the center with popsicle sticks; set aside.

2. In a small sauce pan, melt the nut butter, honey and vanilla together over low/medium heat. Stir constantly until you reach a caramel consistency. Remove from heat.

3. Roll each apple in the caramel one at a time, scraping the excess from the bottom. Roll the apple in optional toppings of choice. Place on parchment paper.

4. Place dark chocolate and white chocolate in two separate, small bowls. Microwave 30 second at a time until fully melted, stirring in between. Pour into separate Ziploc bags. Snip a tiny hole in one of the corners and drizzle over the top of your caramel apples.

5. Let cool in fridge 30 minutes before slicing. Enjoy!

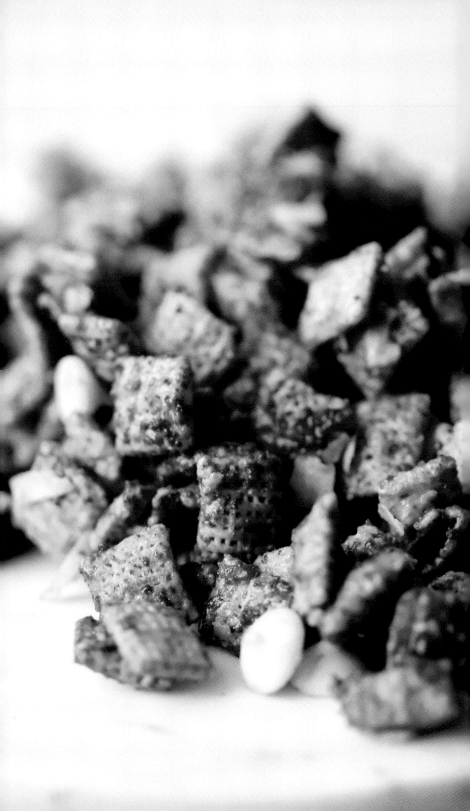

STICKY BUN CHEX MIX

Makes 10 servings
265 calories / 8F / 45.5C / 3P / per serving w/o optional add-ins

3 cups Rice Chex cereal
1 cup Cashew Coconut Caramel Sauce (recipe below)
½ cup coconut sugar
2 tsp. ground cinnamon
Pinch of sea salt
Optional add-ins:
White chocolate chips
Unsweetened flaked coconut
Mini chocolate chips
Chopped pecans or sliced almonds

1. Pour Rice Chex cereal into a large bowl. In a small bowl combine the coconut sugar, cinnamon and sea salt; set aside.

2. Add the caramel sauce to a sauce pan over low heat. Mix until smooth and pourable. Pour over the top of the cereal. Use a large spatula to scrape the sides of the bowl and stir until the cereal is well-coated.

3. Once coated in caramel, pour the cereal into a large Ziploc bag with the sugar/cinnamon mixture. Shake until well-coated. Dump out onto a baking sheet lined with parchment or wax paper. Allow to cool before eating. Enjoy!

CASHEW COCONUT CARAMEL SAUCE
¾ cup salted cashews
¾ cup raw honey
½ cup softened coconut butter (heat in the microwave and stir well)
2-3 Tbs. water
½ tsp. caramel or vanilla extract

1. Soak cashews in water for 1 hour. Drain and place in a high-powered blender with the rest of the ingredients and blend until smooth. Store in the fridge until ready to use.

2. When ready to use, place the caramel sauce in a saucepan over low heat and stir until warm and melted.

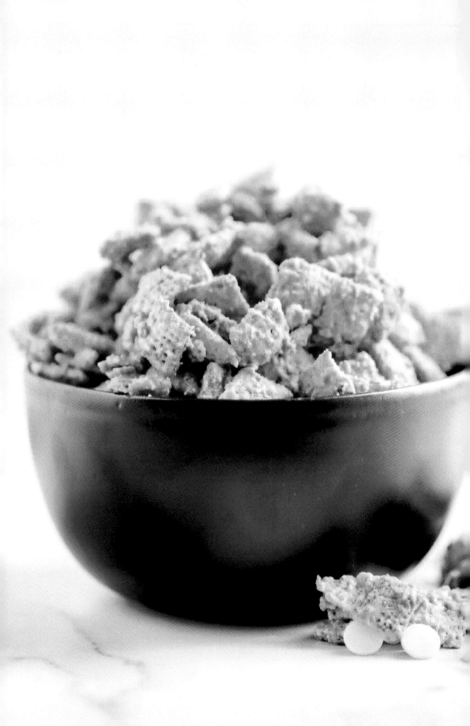

WHITE CHOCOLATE CINNAMON PUPPY CHOW

Makes 16 servings
245 calories / 11F / 29.5C / 6.5P / per serving

3 cups (1 box) Cinnamon Chex cereal
2 Tbs. grass-fed butter
1 cup white chocolate chips
1/2 cup OffBeat Sweet Classic Peanut Butter
    or natural peanut butter
1 serving CSE Simply Vanilla or Snickerdoodle Protein Powder
1/2 cup peanut butter powder

1. Pour Rice Chex cereal into a large bowl.

2. Add the butter, white chocolate chips, and peanut butter to a small saucepan. Melt the ingredients down over low/medium heat. Whisk constantly until smooth and pourable.

3. Pour over the cereal and stir until well coated. Dump into a large Ziploc bag and top with the protein powder and the peanut butter powder. Seal the bag and shake until the cereal is well coated. Pour back into the bowl and enjoy! Store extras in the fridge.

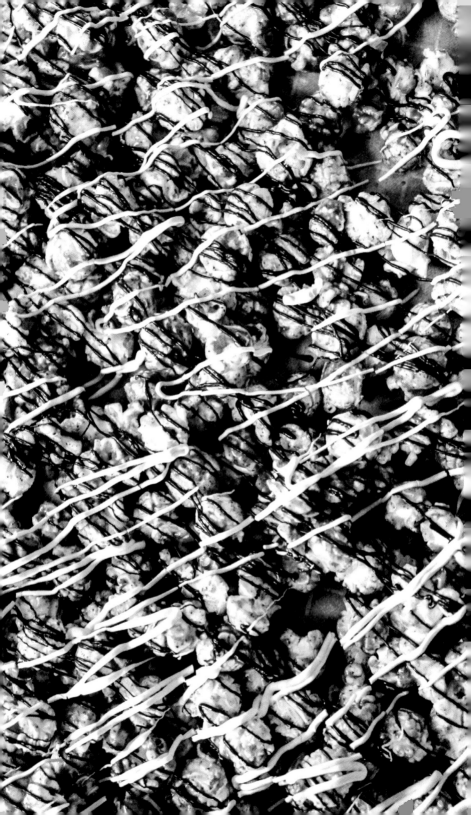

EBRA CARAMEL CORN

Makes 8 servings
265 calories / 11F / 38C / 4P / per serving

12 cups (½ cup kernels) air-popped popcorn
½ cup OffBeat Sweet Classic Peanut Butter, Salted Caramel Butter,
    or natural peanut butter/almond butter
½ cup raw honey
1 tsp. vanilla extract
¼ cup dark chocolate chips
¼ cup white chocolate chips
Pinch of sea salt

1. Pour popped popcorn into a large bowl.

2. In a saucepan, melt the nut butter, honey and vanilla over medium heat. Stir until pourable.

3. Pour over the popcorn and stir until well-coated. Pour out onto a sheet of parchment paper and let cool.

4. In two separate bowls, microwave the chocolate chip flavors, 30 seconds at a time until completely melted and smooth, stirring in between. Pour the dark chocolate into a Ziploc sandwich bag. Cut a small hole in one corner and drizzle over the popcorn. Repeat with the white chocolate. Sprinkle sea salt over the top and store in the fridge to cool.

5. Once the chocolate is hardened, separate into 8 servings. Enjoy!

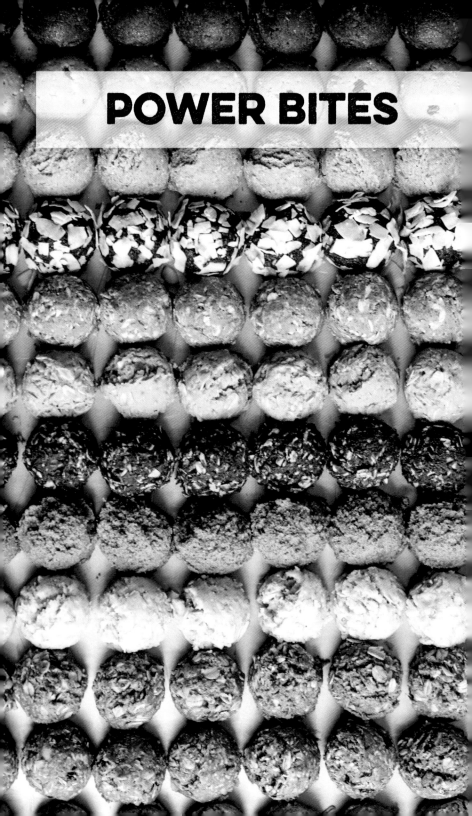

POWER BITES

CELEBRATE THE LITTLE THINGS

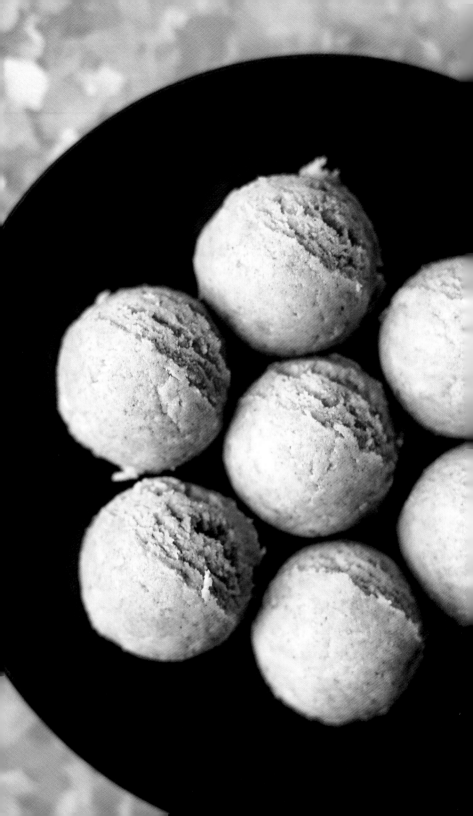

ALMOND FLAX PROTEIN BITES

Makes 36 bites
110 calories / 7F / 7.5C / 4P / per bite

1 cup OffBeat Sweet Classic Peanut Butter, Cinnamon Bun Butter,
    or natural almond butter
½ cup raw honey or pure maple syrup
¼ cup flaxseed meal
2 servings CSE Simply Vanilla Protein Powder
2 tsp. vanilla extract
Dash of sea salt
2 cups almond flour

(Easily prepared in a Kitchen Aid mixer)

1. Mix all the ingredients together, adding the almond flour last, until
well combined.

2. Using a small cookie scoop, scoop into balls and store in the
fridge or freezer. Enjoy!

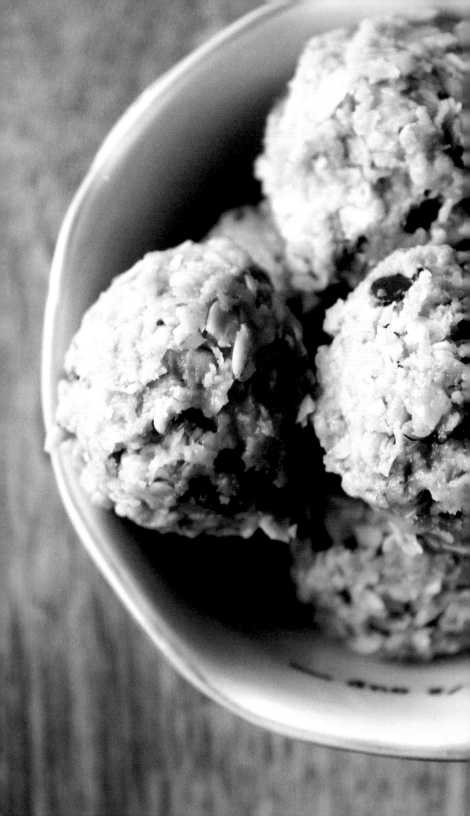

ALMOND JOY COOKIE DOUGH BITES

Makes 32 bites
100 calories / 5F / 11C / 3P / per bite

1/2 cup OffBeat Midnight Almond Coconut Butter
   or natural almond butter
1/2 cup OffBeat Sweet Classic Peanut Butter
   or natural peanut butter
1/2 cup raw honey
1 serving CSE Simply Vanilla or Coconut Cream Protein Powder
1/2 cup unsweetened shredded coconut
1/4 cup flaxseed meal
2 Tbs. cocoa nibs or mini chocolate chips
2 cups old-fashioned rolled oats

(Easily prepared in a Kitchen Aid mixer)

1. Mix all ingredients together, adding the oats last. Mix until well combined.

2. Using a small cookie scoop, scoop into balls and store in the fridge or freezer. Enjoy!

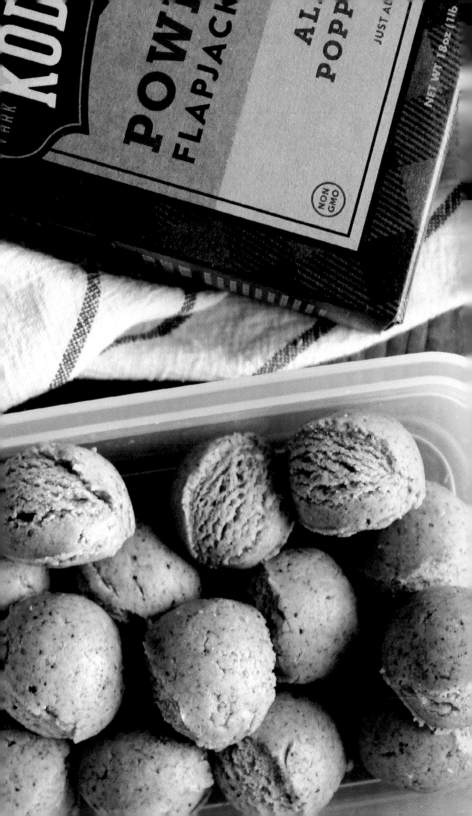

ALMOND POPPY SEED BITES
Makes 30 bites
95 calories / 4.5F / 10C / 4P / per bite

1 cup OffBeat Lemon Coconut Bliss Butter or
  natural almond butter
1/2 cup raw honey
1 serving (33g) CSE Simply Vanilla Protein Powder
1 ½ cups Kodiak Cakes Almond Poppy Seed Mix
Dash sea salt

(Easily prepared in a Kitchen Aid Mixer)

1. Add all of the ingredients to a bowl and mix until well combined.

2. Using a small cookie scoop, scoop into balls and store in the fridge or freezer. Enjoy!

*Consuming raw or undercooked flour may increase your risk of food-borne illness. We recommend cooking the Kodiak Cakes flour mix in the oven at 350 degrees F for at least 5 minutes until the internal temperature of the flour reaches 160 degrees F.

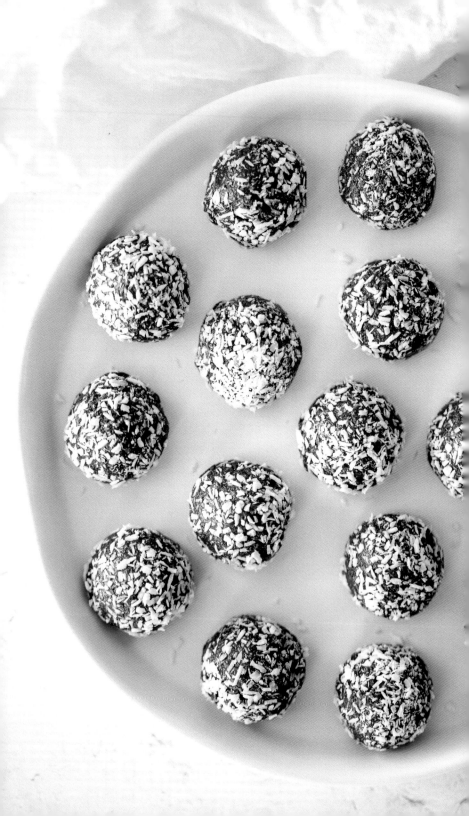

ALMOND COCONUT BROWNIE BITES

Makes 20 bites
105 calories / 5F / 12C / 3.5P / per bite

½ cup OffBeat Midnight Almond Coconut Butter
    or natural almond butter
½ cup raw honey
2 Tbs. coconut oil
1 tsp. almond extract
5 Tbs. cocoa powder
1 serving CSE Brownie Batter or Coconut Cream Protein Powder
¼ cup unsweetened finely shredded coconut
1 cup oat flour

(Easily prepared in a Kitchen Aid mixer)

1. Mix almond butter, honey, coconut oil, almond extract, cocoa powder and protein powder in a bowl. Add oat flour and mix well.

2. Chill in the fridge for at least 30 minutes. Using a small cookie scoop, scoop into balls and roll in shredded coconut. Store in the fridge or freezer. Enjoy!

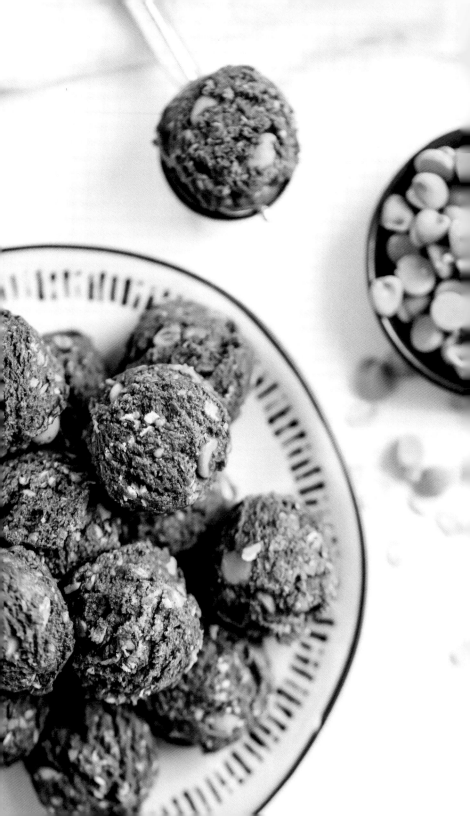

BUCKEYE BROWNIE POWER BITES

Makes 28 bites
110 calories / 5.5F / 12C / 4P / per bite

---

1 cup OffBeat Buckeye Brownie Butter
   or natural peanut butter
1/2 cup raw honey
2 servings CSE Brownie Batter Protein Powder
1 cup old-fashioned rolled oats
1/4 cup Reese's peanut butter chips

(Easily prepared in a Kitchen Aid Mixer)

1. Mix all ingredients together, adding the oats last, until well combined.

2. Using a small cookie scoop, scoop into balls and store in the fridge or freezer. Enjoy!

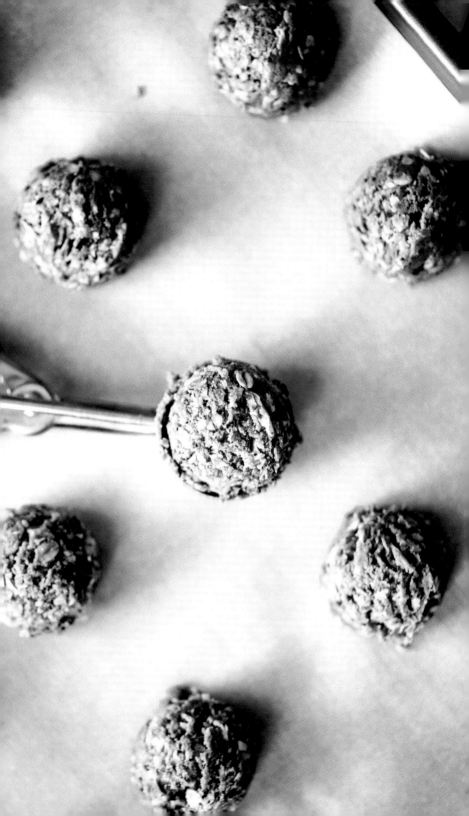

CARAMEL MACCHIATO BITES

Makes 30 bites
90 calories / 4F / 10.5C / 3P / per bite

---

1 cup OffBeat Almond Mocha Butter or
    natural almond butter
½ cup raw honey
2 Tbs. Crio Bru grounds or coffee bean grounds
1 serving CSE Caramel Toffee or Simply Vanilla Protein Powder
½ tsp. vanilla extract
Pinch of sea salt
1 ½ cups old-fashioned rolled oats

(Easily prepared in a Kitchen Aid Mixer)

1. Mix all ingredients together, adding the oats last, until well combined.

2. Using a small cookie scoop, scoop into balls and store in the fridge or freezer. Enjoy!

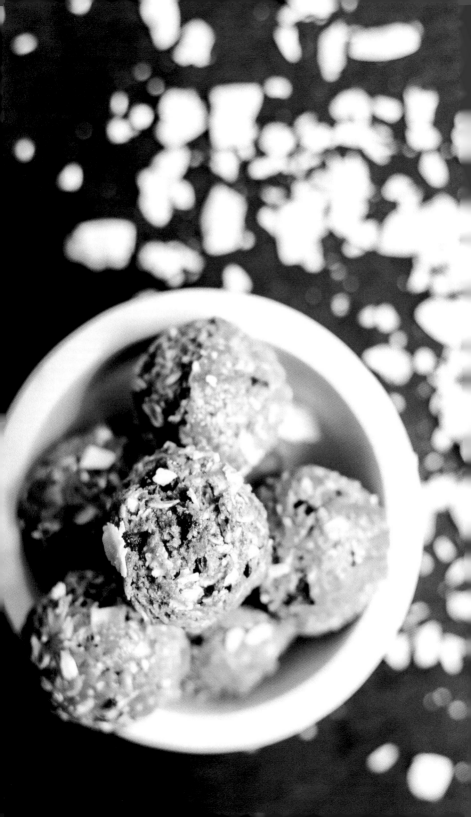

CHOCOLATE ALMOND JOY BITES
Makes 30 bites
100 calories / 5F / 10.5C / 3.5P / per bite

1 cup OffBeat Midnight Almond Coconut Butter or
   natural almond butter
½ cup raw honey
2 servings CSE Brownie Batter Protein Powder
1 Tbs. coconut oil
½ cup unsweetened shredded coconut
2 Tbs. cocoa nibs or mini chocolate chips
1 ½ cups old-fashioned rolled oats
1 tsp. vanilla extract
Dash sea salt

(Easily prepared in a Kitchen Aid Mixer)

1. Mix all ingredients together, adding the oats last, until well combined.

2. Using a small cookie scoop, scoop into balls and store in the fridge or freezer. Enjoy!

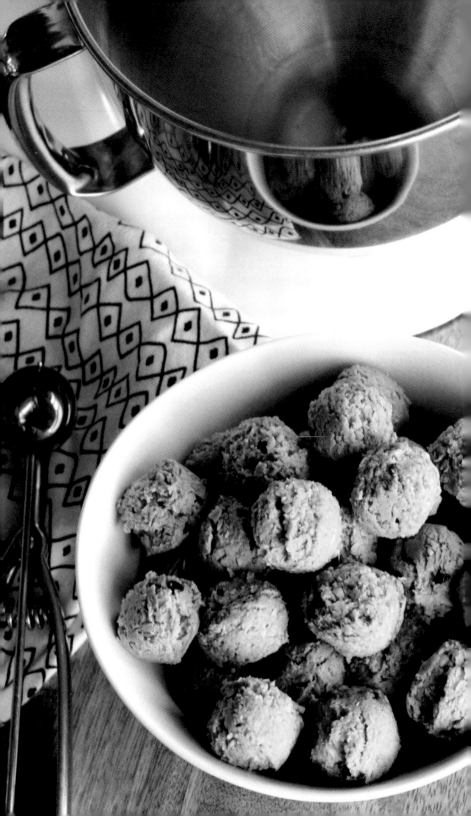

CHOCOLATE CHIP COOKIE DOUGH BITES

Makes 26 bites
105 calories / 5F / 11C / 5P / per bite

___

1 cup OffBeat Sweet Classic Peanut Butter
   or natural peanut butter
1/2 cup raw honey
1 serving CSE Simply Vanilla Protein Powder
1 1/2 cups Kodiak Power Cakes Mix
1 tsp. vanilla extract
Dash of sea salt
30 dark chocolate chips

(Easily prepared in a Kitchen Aid mixer)

1. Mix peanut butter, honey, protein powder, Kodiak Cakes Mix, vanilla and salt together in a large bowl. Stir in the chocolate chips last.

2. Using a cookie scoop, scoop into balls. Store in the fridge or freezer. Enjoy!

*Consuming raw or undercooked flour may increase your risk of food-borne illness. We recommend cooking the Kodiak Cakes flour mix in the oven at 350 degrees F for at least 5 minutes until the internal temperature of the flour reaches 160 degrees F.

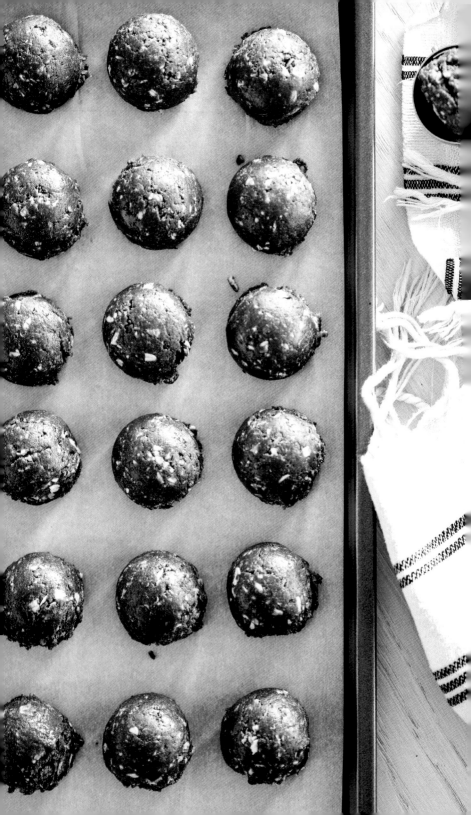

CHOCOLATE PEANUT BUTTER CUP BITES

Makes 34 bites
100 calories / 5F / 11C / 3.5P / per bite

---

12 oz. OffBeat Buckeye Brownie Peanut Butter
   or natural peanut butter
½ cup raw honey
1 serving CSE Brownie Batter or Chocolate Peanut Butter Protein
   Powder
1 cup old-fashioned rolled oats
½ cup Kodiak Cakes Buttermilk Mix
Dash of sea salt
Dash of vanilla extract

(Easily prepared in a Kitchen Aid mixer)

1. Place the peanut butter in the microwave for 30 seconds to soften.
Then scoop into a large bowl. Add remaining ingredients and mix
until well combined.

2. Using a small cookie scoop, scoop into balls and store in the
fridge or freezer. Enjoy!

*Sub more rolled oats for Kodiak Cakes if needed.

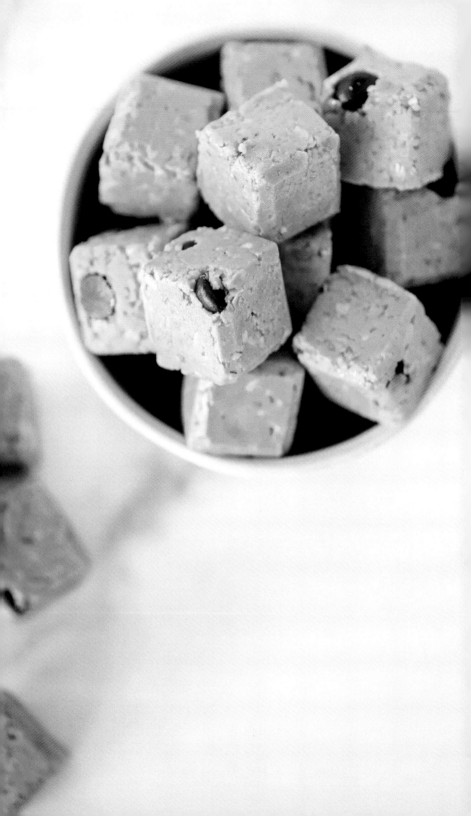

CHUNKY MONKEY BITES

Makes 26 bites
105 calories / 5.5F / 10C / 4.5P / per bite

---

1 cup OffBeat Sweet Classic Peanut Butter, Monkey Business Butter,
   or natural peanut butter
1/2 cup raw honey
2 servings CSE Bananas Foster Protein Powder
1 cup old-fashioned rolled oats
2 Tbs. dark chocolate chips
1/2 tsp. vanilla extract
Pinch of sea salt

(Easily prepared in a Kitchen Aid mixer)

1. Add all the ingredients to a bowl and mix until well combined.

2. Roll into balls or press into an ice cube tray, and place in a
container. Store in the fridge or freezer. Enjoy!

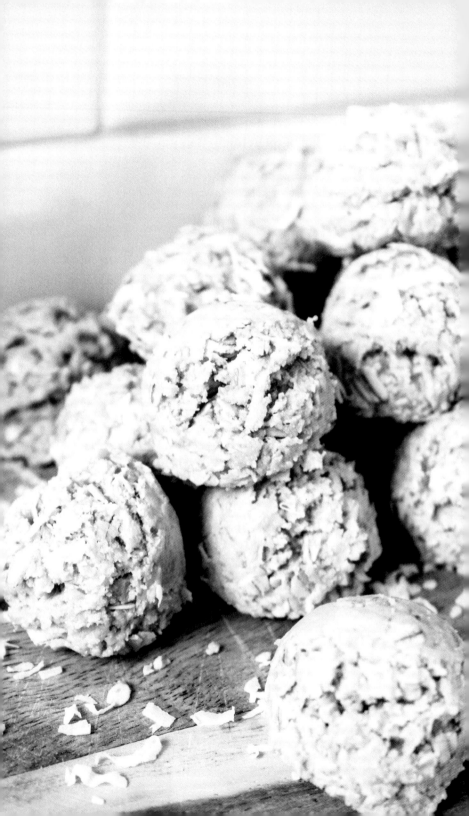

COCONUT CASHEW MACAROON BITES

Makes 35 bites
90 calories / 4.5F / 10C / 3P / per bite

1 cup OffBeat Aloha Butter or
    Toasted Coconut Cashew Butter (recipe below)
½ cup raw honey
2 servings CSE Simply Vanilla or Coconut Cream Protein Powder
½ cup unsweetened coconut flakes
1 tsp. vanilla extract
Pinch of sea salt
2 cups old-fashioned rolled oats

(Easily prepared in a Kitchen Aid mixer)

1. Mix all ingredients together, adding the oats last, until well combined.

2. Using a small cookie scoop, scoop into balls and store in the fridge or freezer. Enjoy!

TOASTED COCONUT CASHEW BUTTER

Makes 1 cup / 16 servings
100 calories / 8.5F / 5C / 3P / per Tbs.

280g roasted, salted cashews
60g unsweetened coconut flakes

1. Place cashews and coconut into a blender and blend until smooth, scraping down the sides in between blends if needed. Pour into a jar or container and store in the fridge.

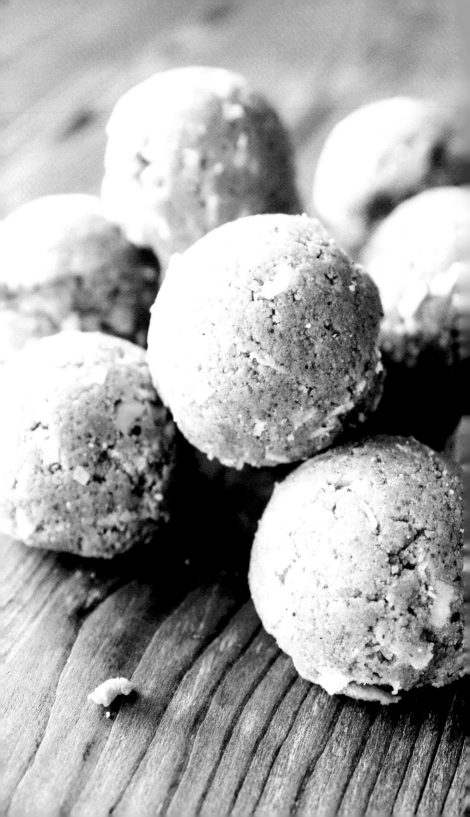

COCONUTTY CINNAMON OAT BITES

Makes 32 bites
100 calories / 5F / 10C / 4P / per bite

½ cup OffBeat Sweet Classic Peanut Butter or
   natural peanut butter
½ cup OffBeat Cinnamon Bun Butter or
   natural almond butter
½ cup raw honey
1 serving CSE Simply Vanilla Protein Powder
1 tsp. vanilla extract
Pinch of sea salt
1 ¼ cups Kodiak Cakes Cinnamon Oat Mix
⅓ cup unsweetened, shredded coconut

(Easily prepared in a Kitchen Aid Mixer)

1. Mix nut butters, honey, protein powder, vanilla and salt together.
Mix in Kodiak Cakes and coconut last.

2. Using a small cookie scoop, scoop into balls and store in the
fridge or freezer. Enjoy!

*Consuming raw or undercooked flour may increase your risk of
food-borne illness. We recommend cooking the Kodiak Cakes flour
mix in the oven at 350 degrees F for at least 5 minutes until the internal temperature of the flour reaches 160 degrees F.

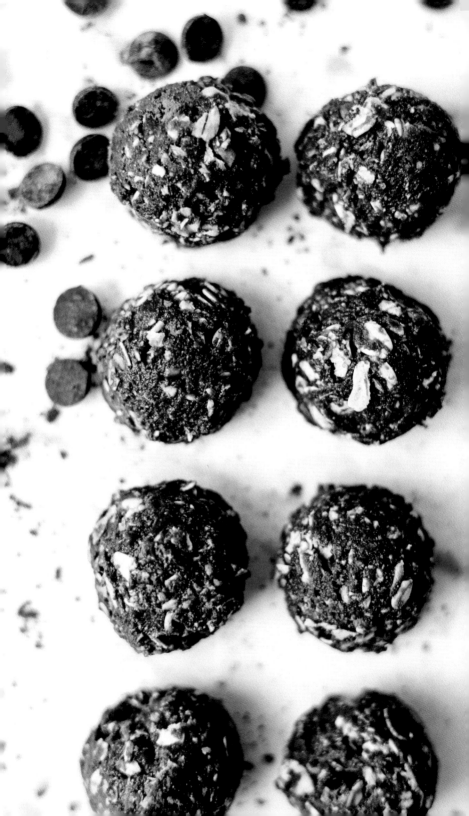

DARK CHOCOLATE PEANUT BUTTER BITES

Makes 26 bites
105 calories / 5.5F / 11.5C / 4P / per bite

1 cup OffBeat Sweet Classic Peanut Butter,
    Buckeye Brownie Peanut Butter, or natural peanut butter
½ cup raw honey
1 serving CSE Brownie Batter or Chocolate Peanut Butter
    Protein Powder
1 ½ cups old-fashioned rolled oats
2 Tbs. cocoa powder
30 extra dark chocolate chips

(Easily prepared in a Kitchen Aid mixer)

1. Mix peanut butter, honey, protein powder, oats and cocoa powder. Stir in chocolate chips last.

2. Using a small cookie scoop, scoop into balls. Store in the fridge or freezer. Enjoy!

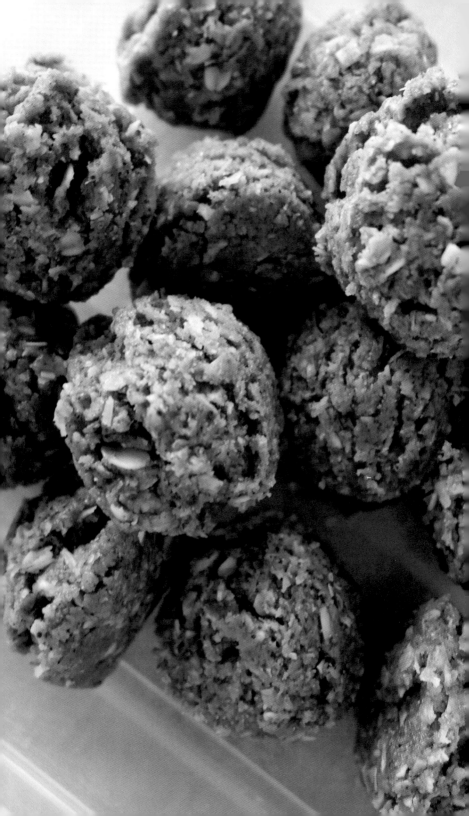

FALL COOKIE DOUGH BITES
Makes 28 bites
100 calories / 5F / 11C / 4P / per bite

---

cup OffBeat Cinnamon Bun Butter, Butter Pecan Pie Butter,
  or natural almond butter
½ cup raw honey
tsp. vanilla extract
1½ cups old-fashioned rolled oats
½ tsp. sea salt
½ tsp. ground cinnamon
¼ tsp. ground nutmeg
2 servings CSE Simply Vanilla or Cinnamon Roll Protein Powder

(Easily prepared in a Kitchen Aid mixer)

1. Place all ingredients into a mixing bowl and stir together until well combined.

2. Scoop into balls using a small cookie scoop. Store in the fridge or freezer. Enjoy!

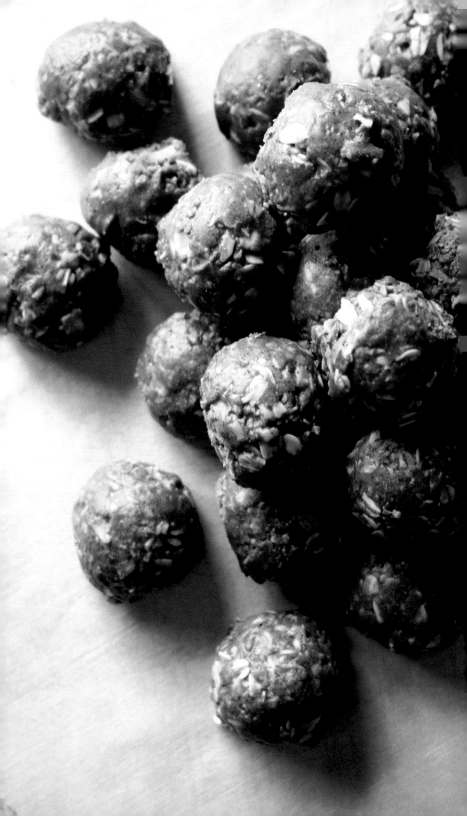

GINGERSNAP ENERGY BITES

Makes 26 bites
15 calories / 7F / 13C / 4P / per bite

¼ cup OffBeat Gingerbread Cookie Butter or
   natural almond butter
¼ cup coconut oil
¼ cup raw honey
¼ cup molasses
   servings CSE Simply Vanilla Protein Powder
   tsp. ground cinnamon
   tsp. ground ginger
½ tsp. vanilla extract
Dash ground cloves
Dash sea salt
2 cups old-fashioned rolled oats

(Easily prepared in a Kitchen Aid mixer)

1. Combine all ingredients except for the oats. Once combined, slowly add in oats. They will be fairly sticky.

2. Using a cookie scoop, scoop into balls and place in a container. Store in fridge to set. Enjoy!

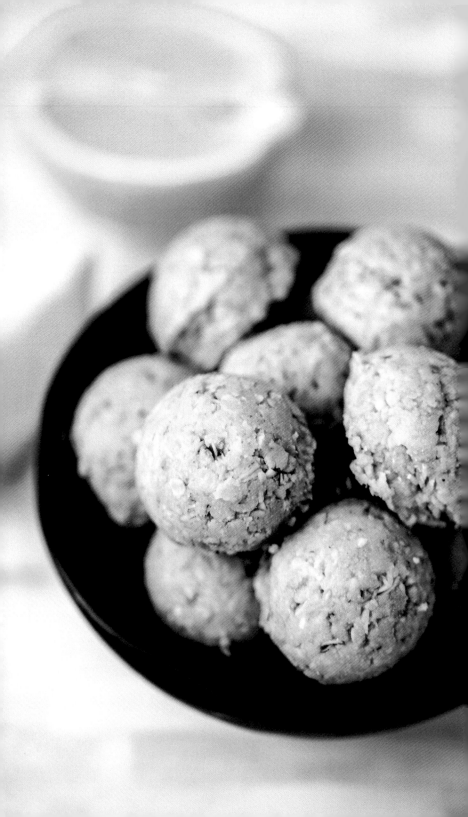

LEMON COCONUT BLISS BITES
Makes 32 bites
100 calories / 6F / 10C / 3P / per bite

cup OffBeat Lemon Coconut Bliss Butter or
  coconut butter, softened
½ cup raw honey
  serving CSE Simply Vanilla or Coconut Cream Protein Powder
¼ cup unsweetened shredded coconut
  Tbs. lemon zest
2 tsp. fresh lemon juice
  tsp. vanilla extract
Pinch of sea salt
1 ½ cups old-fashioned rolled oats

(Easily prepared in a Kitchen Aid mixer)

1. Place all ingredients into a mixing bowl and stir together until well combined.

2. Scoop into balls using a small cookie scoop. Store in the fridge or freezer. Enjoy!

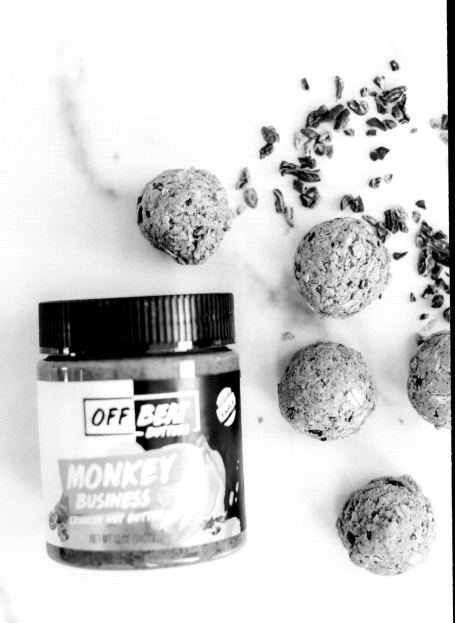

MONKEY BUSINESS BITES

Makes 28 bites
200 calories / 4F / 12C / 4P / per bite

1 cup OffBeat Monkey Business Butter
1/2 cup raw honey
2 servings CSE Bananas Foster, Simply Vanilla,
   or Brownie Batter Protein Powder
1 cup old-fashioned rolled oats
Pinch of coarse sea salt

(Easily prepared in a Kitchen Aid mixer)

1. Place all ingredients into a mixing bowl and stir together until well combined.

2. Scoop into balls using a small cookie scoop. Store in the fridge or freezer. Enjoy!

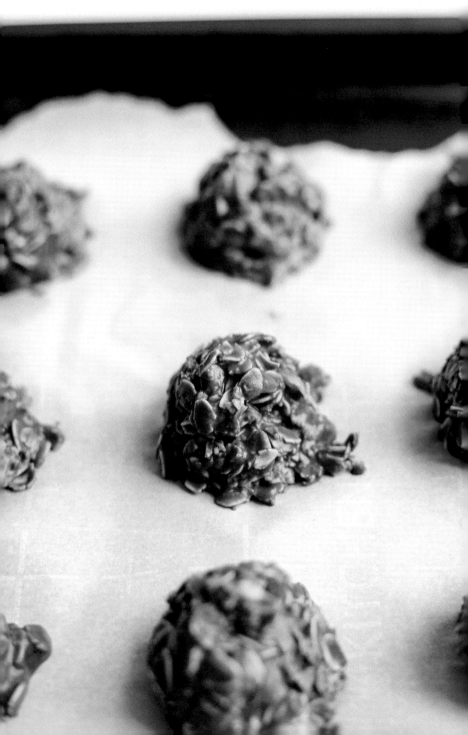

NO-BAKE COOKIE PROTEIN BITES

Makes 28 bites
70 calories / 2F / 10C / 4P / per bite

1½ cups powdered peanut butter
½ cup water
½ cup raw honey
2 Tbs. OffBeat Sweet Classic Peanut Butter
  or natural peanut butter
2 Tbs. melted coconut oil or grass-fed butter
1 serving CSE Brownie Batter or Chocolate Peanut Butter
  Protein Powder
2 Tbs. cocoa powder
½ tsp. vanilla extract
Dash of sea salt
1½ cups old-fashioned rolled oats

(Easily prepared in a Kitchen Aid mixer)

1. Stir powdered peanut butter and water together in a bowl. Stir in all other ingredients until well combined.

2. Using a small cookie scoop, scoop onto a baking sheet lined with parchment or wax paper. Place in the freezer. Once set, transfer to a container and store in the fridge or freezer. Enjoy warm or cold!

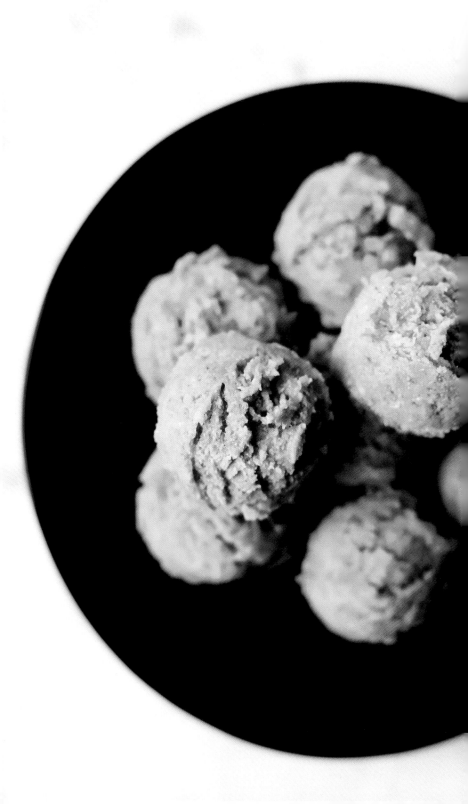

B FIT BITES
Makes 30 bites
70 calories / 1F / 13C / 6P / per bite

1¼ cups powdered peanut butter
½ cup + 2 Tbs. water
1 tsp. vanilla extract
½ cup raw honey
2 servings CSE Simply Vanilla Protein Powder
2 Tbs. mini chocolate chips
½ tsp. sea salt
3 cups Kodiak Cakes Buttermilk Mix

(Easily prepared in a Kitchen Aid mixer)

1. In a large bowl, mix together powdered peanut butter, water, vanilla, honey, protein powder, chocolate chips and sea salt. Add the Kodiak Cakes in last, one cup at a time, until well combined.

2. Using a small cookie scoop, scoop into balls and store in the fridge or freezer. Enjoy!

*Consuming raw or undercooked flour may increase your risk of food-borne illness. We recommend cooking the Kodiak Cakes flour mix in the oven at 350 degrees F for at least 5 minutes until the internal temperature of the flour reaches 160 degrees F.

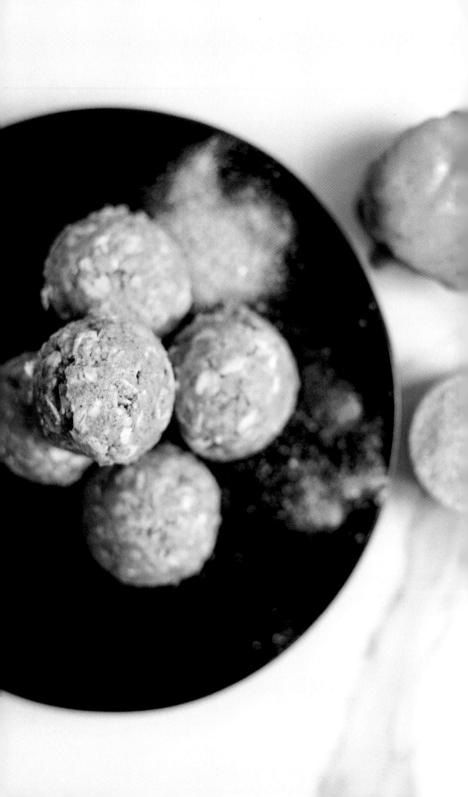

PB&J POWER BITES

Makes 26 bites
75 calories / 3F / 7C / 3P / per bite

---

1 cup OffBeat Sweet Classic Peanut Butter
   or natural peanut butter
½ cup raw honey
2 servings CSE Simply Vanilla or
   Strawberry Cheesecake Protein Powder
2 servings CSE Antioxidants Super Berry Mix
1½ cups old-fashioned rolled oats
Dash vanilla extract
Dash sea salt

(Easily prepared in a Kitchen Aid mixer)

1. Place all ingredients into a mixing bowl and stir together until well combined.

2. Scoop into balls using a small cookie scoop. Store in the fridge or freezer. Enjoy!

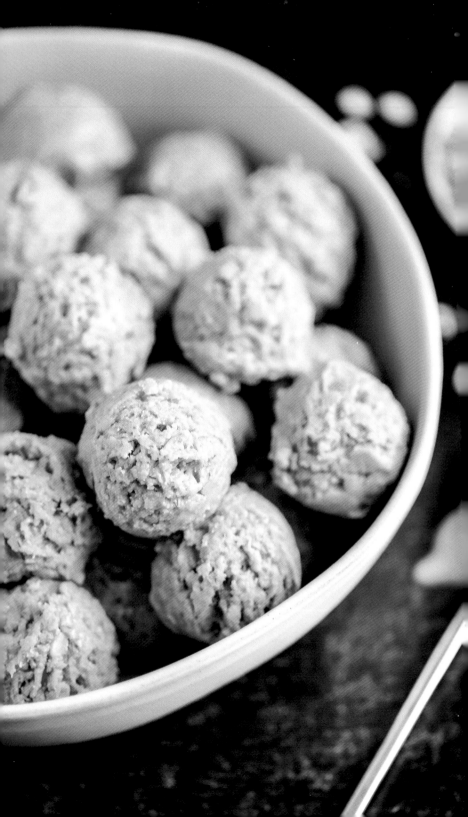

PEANUT BUTTER POWER BITES
Makes 26 bites
90 calories / 5F / 10C / 4P / per bite

---

1 cup OffBeat Sweet Classic Peanut Butter
  or natural peanut butter
½ cup raw honey
2 servings CSE Simply Vanilla Protein Powder
1½ cups old-fashioned rolled oats
Dash vanilla extract
Dash sea salt

(Easily prepared in a Kitchen Aid mixer)

1. Place all ingredients into a mixing bowl and stir together until well combined.

2. Scoop into balls using a small cookie scoop. Store in the fridge or freezer. Enjoy!

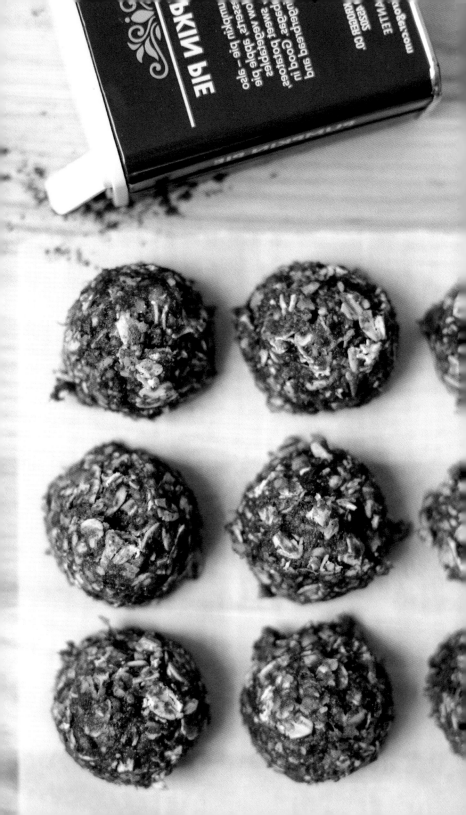

PUMPKIN PIE ENERGY BITES

Makes 32 bites
5 calories / 4F / 9C / 3P / per bite

⅓ cups Medjool dates, pitted
 cup pecans
½ cup unsweetened shredded coconut
½ cup canned pumpkin
 Tbs. vanilla extract
 tsp. ground cinnamon
½ tsp. ground nutmeg
Dash of ground cloves
Dash of sea salt
 servings CSE Simply Vanilla or Pumpkin Pie Protein Powder
 cups old-fashioned rolled oats

(Easily prepared in a Kitchen Aid mixer)

1. Soak dates for 10 minutes. Drain.

2. Place pecans in a food processor or high-powered blender and
pulse until broken up. Add the dates, coconut, pumpkin, vanilla,
spices and salt. Pulse until combined.

3. Transfer to a bowl and stir in protein powder and oats. Store in the
fridge for 30 minutes. Using a cookie scoop, roll into balls and store
in the fridge or freezer. Enjoy!

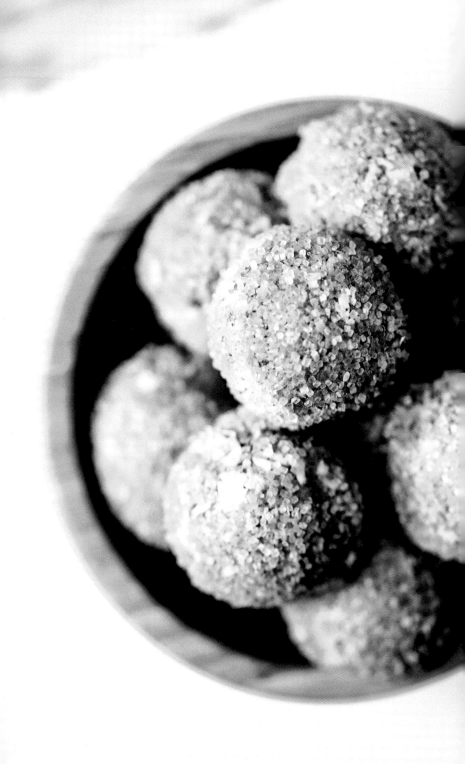

SALTED CARAMEL BITES
Makes 26 bites
100 calories / 5F / 12C / 4P / per bite

---

1 cup OffBeat Salted Caramel Butter
 or natural almond butter
½ cup raw honey
1 serving CSE Simply Vanilla or Caramel Toffee Protein Powder
1½ cups old-fashioned rolled oats
¼ cup Sugar in the Raw or Turbinado Sugar
If using regular almond butter:
1 tsp. caramel extract
Dash coarse sea salt

(Easily prepared in a Kitchen Aid mixer)

1. Add the Salted Caramel Butter or almond butter to a bowl with
the honey, protein powder and rolled oats. Mix until well combined.
If using almond butter instead of the Salted Caramel Butter, stir in
the caramel extract and sea salt.

2. Scoop into balls using a small cookie scoop.

3. Place the sugar into a bowl and roll each ball into the sugar. Place
all of the balls into a container. Store in the fridge or freezer. Enjoy!

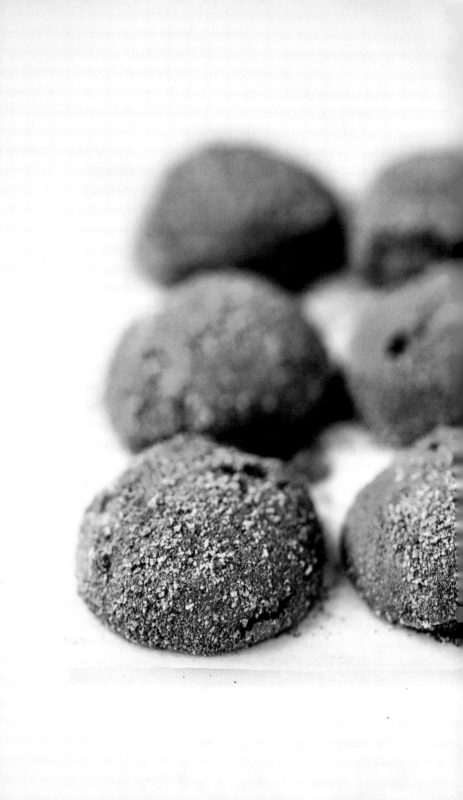

SNICKERDOODLE BITES

Makes 26 bites
100 calories / 4.5F / 12C / 4.5P / per bite

---

1 cup OffBeat Cinnamon Bun Butter
   or natural almond butter
½ cup pure maple syrup
2 servings CSE Simply Vanilla or Snickerdoodle Protein Powder
1½ cups Kodiak Cakes Buttermilk Mix
1 Tbs. ground cinnamon
2 tsp. butter extract
2 tsp. vanilla extract
½ tsp. sea salt

Optional Topping:
1 Tbs. Truvia
½ Tbs. cinnamon

(Easily prepared in a Kitchen Aid mixer)

1. Add the Cinnamon Bun Butter or almond butter to a bowl with the pure maple syrup, protein powder, Kodiak Cakes, cinnamon, butter extract, vanilla extract and sea salt.

2. Scoop into balls using a small cookie scoop.

3. Place the Truvia and cinnamon in a small bowl and roll each ball into the mixture. Place all of the balls into a container. Store in the fridge or freezer. Enjoy!

*Consuming raw or undercooked flour may increase your risk of food-borne illness. We recommend cooking the Kodiak Cakes flour mix in the oven at 350 degrees F for at least 5 minutes until the internal temperature of the flour reaches 160 degrees F.

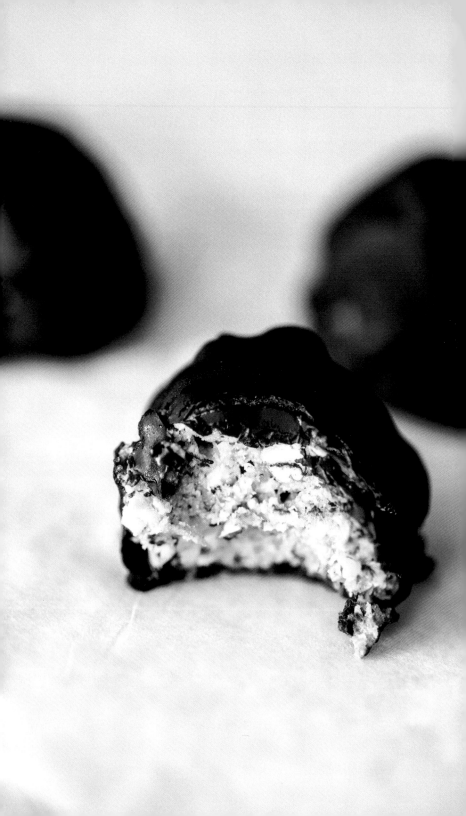

SNICKERS POWER BITES

Makes 28 bites

Macros with the cocoa dusting:
  100 calories / 5F / 10.5C / 4P per serving

Macros with the chocolate coating:
  110 calories / 5.5F / 11C / 4P / per serving

---

1 cup OffBeat Candy Bar Peanut Butter, OffBeat Sweet Classic
  Peanut Butter, OffBeat Salted Caramel Butter,
  or natural peanut butter
½ cup raw honey
1 serving CSE Caramel Toffee, Chocolate Peanut Butter
  or Simply Vanilla Protein Powder
½ tsp. vanilla extract
Dash of sea salt
1½ cups old-fashioned rolled oats

Cocoa Dusting
¼ cup cocoa powder

Chocolate Coating
120g dark chocolate chips

(Easily prepared in a Kitchen Aid mixer)

1. Add all the ingredients to a large bowl and mix until well combined.

2. Using a small cookie scoop, scoop into balls.

3A. If using the Cocoa Dusting method: Add the cocoa powder to a bowl and roll each ball into it. Place in a container and store in the fridge or freezer.

3B. If using the Chocolate Coating method: Add the chocolate chips to a microwave safe bowl. Microwave in 30 second increments, stirring after each one, until melted and smooth.

4. Roll each ball in the chocolate coating and scoop out using a fork or slotted spoon. Tap on bowl to remove excess chocolate then place on a baking sheet lined with parchment paper. Place in the fridge or freezer to allow the chocolate coating to set. Transfer to a container and store in the fridge or freezer.

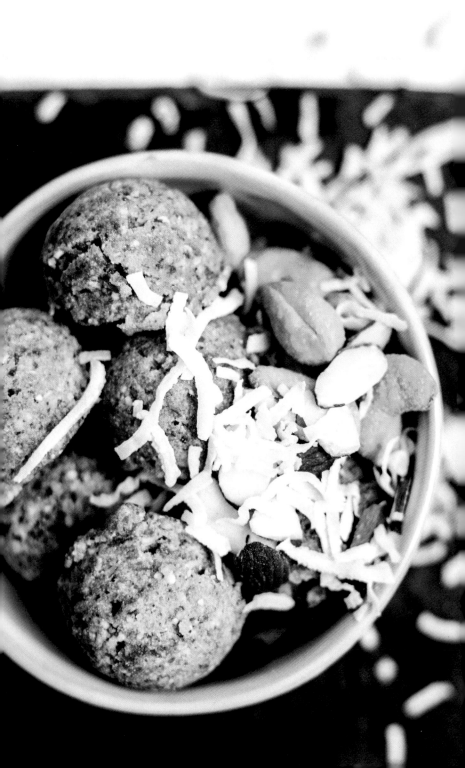

SWEET COCONUTTY ENERGY BITES

Makes 20 bites
90 calories / 6F / 11C / 3P / per bite

---

1 cup almonds
1 cup cashews
1 cup unsweetened shredded coconut
1/2 cups dates, pitted
1 Tbs. coconut oil
1 serving CSE Simply Vanilla
   or Coconut Cream Protein Powder
Dash sea salt

(Easily prepared in a Kitchen Aid mixer)

1. Add almonds, cashews and coconut to a food processor or high-powered blender. Pulse until nuts are finely chopped. Add dates and coconut oil. Pulse until dates are finely chopped and mixture begins to stick together. Stir in protein powder and sea salt; Mix well.

2. Scoop into balls using a small cookie scoop. Store in the fridge or freezer. Enjoy!

If too crumbly, add a little bit of almond milk to form.

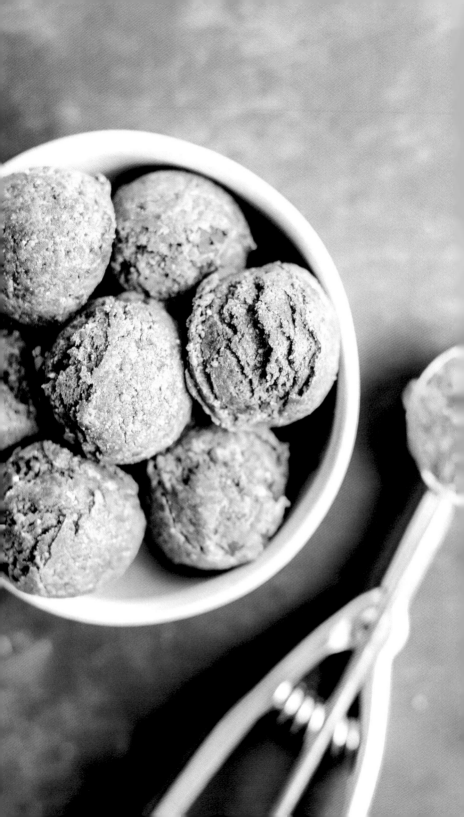

HIN MINT COOKIE BITES

akes 34 bites

calories / 3.5F / 12.5C / 4P / per bite

---

oz. OffBeat Mint Chocolate Chip Cookie Butter
cup raw honey
servings CSE Brownie Batter or Mint Chocolate Cookie
Protein Powder
2 cups Kodiak Cakes Buttermilk Mix
ash vanilla extract
ash sea salt

asily prepared in a Kitchen Aid mixer)

Place all ingredients into a mixing bowl and stir together until well
ombined.

Scoop into balls using a small cookie scoop. Store in the fridge or
eezer. Enjoy!

Consuming raw or undercooked flour may increase your risk of
od-borne illness. We recommend cooking the Kodiak Cakes flour
ix in the oven at 350 degrees F for at least 5 minutes until the inter-
al temperature of the flour reaches 160 degrees F.

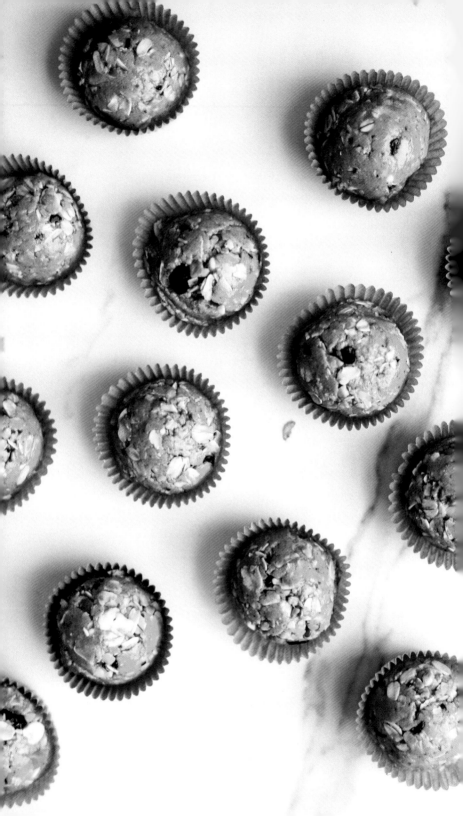

TRIPLE-CHIP BUTTERSCOTCH BITES

Makes 30 bites
90 calories / 5F / 10.5C / 4P / per serving

---

1 cup OffBeat Sweet Classic Peanut Butter
or natural peanut butter
1 cup raw honey
1 tsp. vanilla extract
2 servings CSE Simply Vanilla Protein Powder
1½ cups old-fashioned rolled oats
dash of sea salt
1 Tbs. chopped butterscotch chips
1 Tbs. chopped dark chocolate chips
1 Tbs. chopped white chocolate chips

(easily prepared in a Kitchen Aid mixer)

1. Add the peanut butter, honey and vanilla to a bowl and mix well.

2. In a separate bowl, combine the protein powder, oats, sea salt and all the chocolate chips. Add the wet ingredients to the dry ingredients; mix until well combined.

3. Using a cookie small scoop, scoop into balls and place in a container. Store in the fridge or freezer.

CLEAN
SIMPLE
SWAPS

WHITE WHOLE WHEAT FLOUR OR KODIAK CAKES BUTTERMILK MIX BAKING MIX	KODIAK CAKES GLUTEN-FREE MIX, BOB'S RED MILL GLUTEN-FREE ALL-PURPOSE BAKING FLOUR, KING ARTHUR GLUTEN-FREE FLOUR OR ALL-PURPOSE MIX OR THRIVE MARKET PALEO FLOUR
GRASS-FED BUTTER	COCONUT OIL
DARK CHOCOLATE CHIPS	ENJOY LIFE CHOCOLATE CHIPS OR NESTLE TOLL-HOUSE SIMPLY DELICIOUS SEMI-SWEET MORSELS
WHITE CHOCOLATE CHIPS	KING DAVID WHITE CHOCO CHIPS C ARTISAN KETTLE WHITE CHOCOLAT CHIPS
GREEK YOGURT	PLAIN KITE HILL ALMOND MILK YOGURT, PLAIN FORAGER CASHEW-GURT OR PLAIN SO DELICIOUS COCONUT MILK YOGURT
CREAM CHEESE	TRADER JOE'S VEGAN CREAM CHEESE OR DAIYA CREAM CHEESE STYLE SPREAD
WHIPPED CREAM OR REDDI WIP	ALMOND MILK REDDI WIP OR COCONUT MILK REDDI WIP
CARAMEL FLAVORED CHIPS	KING DAVID VEGAN CARAMEL CHIPS
BUTTERSCOTCH CHIPS	KING DAVID BUTTERSCOTCH CHIPS
BUTTER EXTRACT	VANILLA OR ALMOND EXTRACT
FAT-FREE MILK	CASHEW MILK, COCONUT MILK OR ALMOND MILK
WHEY PROTEIN POWDER	CSE VEGAN PROTEIN POWDER

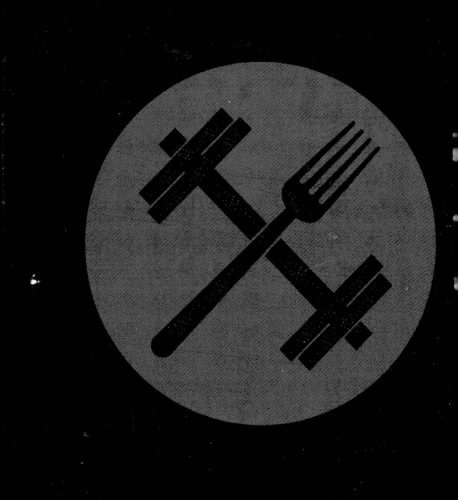